I0146387

Macro Diet

Recipes

1001

Days Easy & Healthy Recipes and Example Food Plan to Help you Burn Fat Fast

© Copyright 2021 by **Virginia Harris**

Table of Contents

Warnings

The following indications have an EXCLUSIVE informative purpose and are not intended to replace the opinion of professional figures such as doctors, nutritionists or dieticians, whose intervention is necessary for the prescription and composition of PERSONALIZED food therapies.

Macrobiotic Diet

The macrobiotic diet is a dietary regimen that proposes a vision of food as a deep nutrient following the alternation of Yin and Yang.

"Philosophy of macrobiotics

If we wanted to explain it in biochemical terms, we could say that yin corresponds to an acidic pH (acidifying foods) and yang to a basic one (alkalizing foods), but we do not always find this kind of coincidence.

It can be considered a technique of personal evolution, in the same way as yoga, Japanese budō in its essence or the various spiritual disciplines.

According to George Ohsawa - ambassador of the macrobiotic diet from Japan to the European continent - the balance of the human organism would be of five Yin to one Yang (this relationship would correspond to that of the presence of sodium -Yin- and potassium -Yang- in the composition of our blood).

Main foods

To practice macrobiotics one must first learn about food. Discovering whole foods is essential to begin entering the world of macrobiotics. Each whole food is a unique combination of natural vitamins, trace elements, unsaturated fatty acids, biostimoline. In macrobiotic cooking, rather than chemically processed substances that alter the digestive process, we prefer natural foods that come from crops characterized by the use of organic fertilizers and the exclusion of chemical fertilizers, herbicides and toxic fungicides. Individual foods can be classified in yin and yang foods. It is a very complex distinction, which has its roots in Taoist philosophy; to use a famous phrase by George Oshawa, "Yin and Yang are the hands of the universe". In a very summary way we can say that yang foods contain more sodium, have a salty, not very sweet or spicy taste and higher degree of alkalinity; whereas yin foods contain more potassium, have a sweet or spicy taste and higher degree of acidity. Many times this distinction is overlooked and people mistakenly think that macrobiotic cooking is just a variation of vegetarian. In reality, macrobiotics does not exclude the occasional consumption of fish and other organisms of marine origin. Besides cereals, legumes and vegetables, typical foods of macrobiotic tradition include miso (made of fermented soy and cereals), soy sauce, tofu (soy cheese), seaweeds and preserved roots. The preferred cooking methods are steaming or baking and if foods must be sweetened, cane sugar or sweet compounds such as maple or rice syrup are used; instead of coffee and tea it is preferred to consume green tea or barley coffee.

Benefits and contraindications of macrobiotic diet

The macrobiotic diet has the merit of having made known to the whole world foods of oriental taste and origin with remarkable healing properties, such as seaweeds. It is an excellent diet for those who want to reduce cholesterol or eliminate toxins. The real problematic aspect of this diet is that it is based on a very precise philosophy, which the one who starts walking towards a macrobiotic path must have first assimilated, made it his or her own, as much as possible. Often one meets with deficiencies or imbalances because one neglects or underestimates the fundamental principle of balance, be it between yin and yang foods, be it in life and in the decisions on which it is articulated.

The meaning of macrobiotic diet: health and balance

The macrobiotic diet strongly opposes the consumption of sophisticated and preserved foods, sugars and sweets, and promotes instead the consumption of vegetables, except for tomatoes, potatoes, eggplants and peppers, which belong to the family of solanaceous plants, therefore being strongly acidifying. The supporters of macrobiotics in fact pursue health through the achievement of the balance between Yin and Yang, between acid and alkaline. The macrobiotic diet then, excludes all animal proteins (meat, fish, milk and derivatives): in a soft macrobiotic diet is allowed the consumption of fish.

Chewing water and drinking food

The assertion "chew water and drink food" is one of the first teachings of macrobiotics, and means that water should not be swallowed quickly and that food should be chewed enough to become liquid. This method serves to facilitate digestion, keeping in mind that starches present in cereals are digested by means of amylase, an enzyme produced in the mouth during chewing which allows the assimilation of starches.

How to balance foods in the diet: examples

In order not to involve dietary deficiency risks, a macrobiotic diet must include the following foods:

~ whole grains: rice, oats, barley, wheat, buckwheat, corn, rye, millet, quinoa, amaranth;
~ vegetables and algae (the latter for their high protein value);
~ legumes: lentils, chickpeas, beans, peas, soybeans or derivatives such as tofu;
~ Kombu, wakame, Nori and Hiziki seaweeds;
~ fresh fruit in season, consumed away from meals and one type at a time;
~ seeds, nuts, spices, black and white sesame seeds, sunflower seeds, pumpkin seeds, peanuts, hazelnuts, walnuts, chestnuts and almonds;
~ in moderation, sea salt, ginger, mustard seeds, apple cider vinegar, garlic, lemon and apple juice.

Pros and cons of macrobiotic diet

As it is a diet without therapeutic indications, it should be considered that, if prolonged for years, the adoption of the macrobiotic diet in the strict sense can induce an iron deficiency because of the consumption of cereals and the presence of phytic acid. The use of seaweeds can partially compensate this "defect".

Example of macrobiotic diet: dish composition

An example of a complete dish with the macrobiotic diet could be composed in this way:

~ 50% whole grains in unrefined grains such as long grain rice and basmati rice, barley, millet, spelt wheat, buckwheat, corn, oats
~ 20% to 30% raw and cooked seasonal vegetables such as all types of cabbage, carrots, fennel, zucchini and green beans
~ 10% to 20% of proteins such as fish, seitan, feta cheese, soy steaks and legumes such as lentils, peas, chickpeas, soy, Azuki (Japanese red beans)
~ 10% fresh or dried fruit or seaweed (Wakame, Kombu) or sweets without sugar or dairy products

Rules of Macrobiotic Cuisine

To choose the best foods it is necessary

~ avoid overly processed or refined foods, vegetables grown with the use of chemical additives, consumption of meat or eggs from animals fed with feed containing additives, consumption of milk and dairy products, frozen vegetables, shellfish, exotic fruits, potatoes, tomatoes, mushrooms and eggplant;
~ eliminate coffee, honey and sugar and all foods containing them;
~ consume more fish;
~ chew for a long time.

Menu and glossary of foods present in the macrobiotic diet

Seitan: wheat gluten processed and cooked in soy sauce: cannot be used by those who are intolerant to gluten, high protein, excellent substitute for meat, useful for stews and fake roasts.

Tofu: processing with the addition of rennet to soy milk in order to obtain a false cheese, also of protein nature.

Toasted Bancha: tea of Japanese origin (camellia sinensis) rich in calcium, excellent for breakfast.

Tea mu: compote of energetic tonic roots. To drink during the day.

Shoyu and tamari: fermented soy sauces useful as condiment and to improve digestion.

Umeboshi: salty and acid digestive alkalizing plums.

Kuzu: starch of burdock root, cleanser and re-balancer of the intestine.

All of the above foods are available in herbalist stores and in the best organic supermarkets.

Starters

Quick savouries

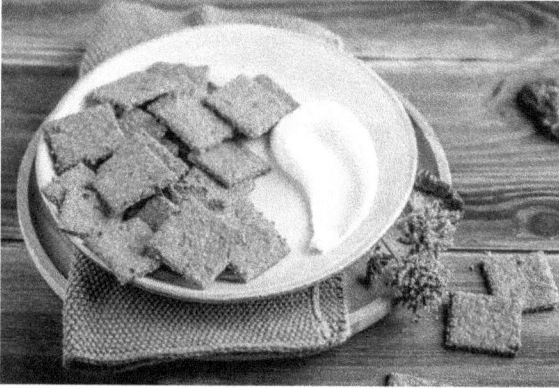

Ingredients

For the dough:

~ 150 g semi-whole wheat flour type 1 or type 2 or whole wheat flour
~ 50 g of evo oil
~ ½ teaspoon of integral sea salt
~ water

For seasoning

~ oregano and paprika (or other flavourings as desired)
~ salt or soy sauce

Instructions

Mix the flour with salt and oil. Add a little water to mix and obtain a compact but soft dough. If you have time, make a ball, wrap it in plastic wrap and let it rest in the refrigerator for half an hour. Otherwise immediately roll out the dough with a rolling pin leaving it to a thickness of about 2-3 millimetres. Roll out the dough on greaseproof paper so that the savouries are ready to be baked.

Season to taste with salt or brush with soy sauce. Add the flavours of your choice. I added oregano and paprika, but you can use curry, turmeric, various finely chopped flavourings, poppy seeds, etc.

Cut the dough with a pizza wheel or knife, shaping the pretzels any way you like. Move the baking paper with the pretzels on top to a baking sheet and bake at 350 degrees for about 10 minutes.

Crunchy chickpea snacks

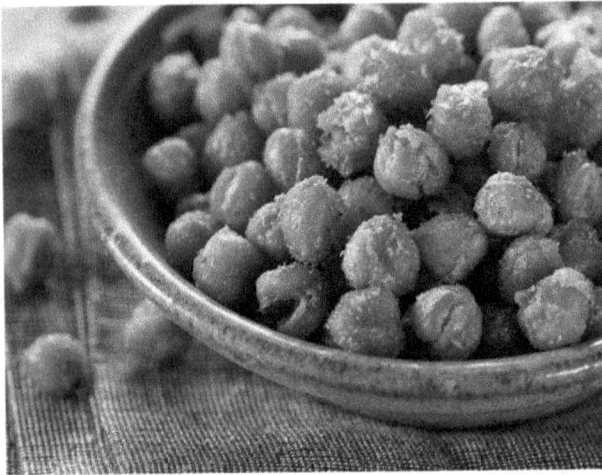

around. At this point bake for 1 hour. Total cooking time is 1 1/2 hours.

Ingredients

- ~ 200 g of boiled chickpeas
- ~ 1 tablespoon of oregano
- ~ 1 teaspoon of whole sea salt
- ~ 1/2 teaspoon of sweet curry
- ~ 1 pinch of ground cumin
- ~ 1 handful of almonds reduced to flour
- ~ 2 tablespoons extra virgin olive oil

Instructions

Heat oven to 180 degrees. In the meantime, dry the chickpeas well and remove the skins by rubbing them. It 'an operation that requires a little patience, but it is essential to make the sauce stick better. Transfer them to a bowl and mix well with the oil. In a separate bowl mix the spices, salt and almond flour. Add the chickpeas and mix well.

Place the chickpeas on a baking sheet covered with parchment paper and spread them out so that they do not overlap. Bake and lower the temperature to 150°. Cook 30 minutes then shake the baking sheet to move the chickpeas

Speedy Amaranth with Mediterranean sauce

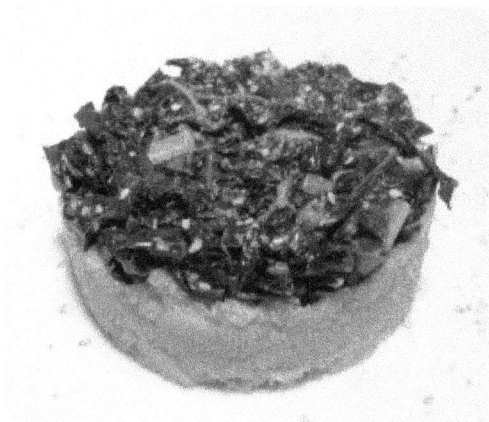

In the meantime, transfer all the ingredients for the sauce to a blender and blend well. Add a little water if necessary. If you don't like to feel the almond bits under your teeth, you can chop the almonds separately, reducing them to flour and add them to the mixture.

Combine the amaranth with the sauce and mix well.

Ingredients

- ~ 1 cup of amaranth (130-150 g)
- ~ 1 pinch of whole sea salt
- ~ For the sauce:
- ~ about 20 g capers
- ~ about 40 g of almonds
- ~ about 20 g of raisins
- ~ 1 small garlic clove (optional)
- ~ 2 fresh tomatoes
- ~ 4-5 tablespoons of extra virgin olive oil
- ~ water (but you may not need it)
- ~ 4-5 basil leaves

For presentation:

- ~ cherry tomatoes (or lettuce leaves)
- ~ basil leaves

Instructions

Put the amaranth in a pot with 2 cups of water and a pinch of salt. Bring to a boil and cook covered for 10-15 minutes. At the end of cooking turn off and let rest covered 10 minutes.

Seaweed pate

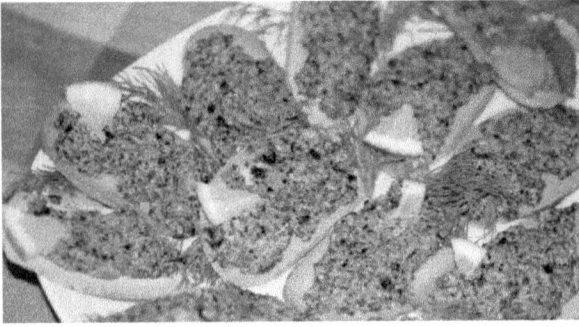

Combine the onions with the seaweed and chop or blend in a blender.

You can spread the pate on croutons and garnish with sesame seeds or use it as a pasta or boiled cereal topping.

Ingredients

~ 1 handful (about 5-6 g) of hiziki seaweed
~ 1 handful (about 5-6 g) of arame seaweed
~ 3 tablespoons olive oil or sesame oil
~ 3-4 tablespoons tamari or shoyu (soy sauce)
~ 2 tablespoons of rice or apple cider vinegar acidulate
~ 1 clove of garlic, minced
~ 1 onion, chopped
~ 700 ml water

Instructions

Soak the seaweed for 15 minutes.

Sauté garlic and onion in oil until soft, remove from pan and set aside.

In the same pan, put the seaweed, water, vinegar and soy sauce and bring to a boil.

Cook uncovered over high heat for 20-30 minutes until the water has completely evaporated.

Millet, pumpkin and hazelnut sticks

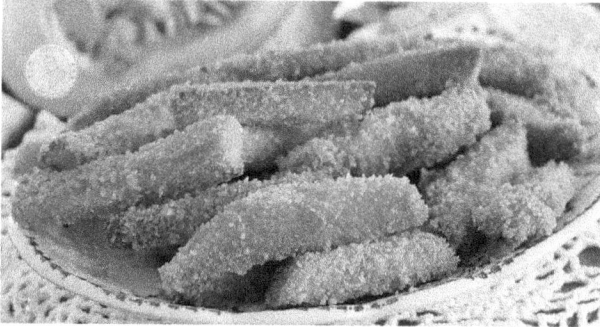

Ingredients

- ~ 100-120 g hulled millet
- ~ 1 onion
- ~ 250 g of cleaned pumpkin
- ~ 3 cabbage leaves
- ~ 1 handful of hazelnuts
- ~ 2 tablespoons extra virgin olive oil or sesame oil
- ~ 2-3 tablespoons of tamari
- ~ whole sea salt
- ~ corn flour
- ~ oil

For the cream:

- ~ 150 g boiled cannellini beans
- ~ 1 scant tablespoon of extra virgin olive oil
- ~ 1 small spoon of tamari
- ~ a few drops of lemon juice (to taste)

Instructions

Wash the millet well and boil it with twice the volume of water and a pinch of salt for about 10 minutes.

The cooking of millet is a bit particular especially because depending on the brands the cooking time changes, varying from 10 to 20 minutes. So the first time you need to experiment.

When cooking takes 10, maximum 15 minutes, double the amount of water is enough, otherwise three times as much is needed.

Bring to a boil, lower the flame to a minimum and put a lid leaving a small gap. After 10 minutes, if the cooking time is correct, the millet will have swollen and the water will be almost completely absorbed. At that point turn it off and let it rest covered for another 10 minutes. Otherwise, add water and continue cooking.

Chop the onion and brown it in a pan with oil and a pinch of salt for a few minutes. In the meantime, dice the pumpkin and add it to the pan with a little water. Continue cooking covered.

Chop the savoy cabbage and the hazelnuts. When the squash is cooked, add the soy sauce, the savoy cabbage and the hazelnuts and continue cooking until the savoy cabbage is cooked, at which point you can add the millet and mix well.

Let cool, then with damp hands form sticks (or whatever shape you prefer) and dip them in the cornmeal. If the dough is too wet and doesn't stay together, you can add some flaked cornmeal to dry it out, then make the sticks and bread them.

Heat a frying pan with a little oil and when it's hot, transfer the sticks and brown them on both sides. If you prefer you can transfer them to a greased baking sheet and bake them for 15 minutes.

Prepare the cannellini cream by blending them well with oil, shoyu and a few drops of lemon.

Serve the sticks accompanied by the cream and a slice of lemon to squeeze over the sticks.

I decorated the cannellini cream with a strip of sweet paprika and the sticks with Zatar, a mixture of oregano, sesame, sumac and salt.

Baked leeks with sweet paprika

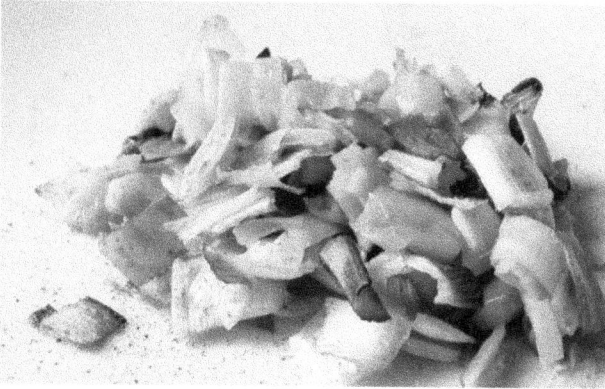

Ingredients

- ~ 2 leeks
- ~ extra virgin olive oil
- ~ 1-2 tablespoons of soy sauce
- ~ paprika to taste

Instructions

Clean and slice the leek as you prefer, into rounds or strips.

Transfer to a baking sheet covered with parchment paper and add oil (I think I put two or three tablespoons in my eyes), then add the soy sauce and paprika and mix with your hands.

Distribute the leeks well throughout the baking dish and bake for about 20 minutes at 180 degrees.

Lentil and Ginger Hummus

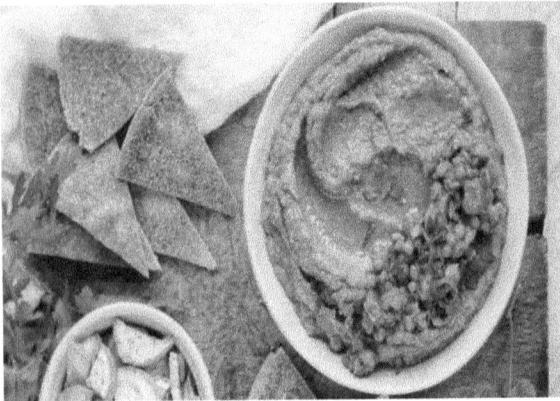

Ingredients

- ~ 200 g cooked lentils (or 80 g dried)
- ~ 2 teaspoons of Shiro miso
- ~ 1 teaspoon of mustard
- ~ 2 tablespoons extra virgin olive oil
- ~ 1 teaspoon or more of ginger juice
- ~ 1 garlic slice (optional)
- ~ 1 teaspoon of shoyu (soy sauce)

Instructions

Blend lentils with all other ingredients and if necessary add water until you get your preferred consistency.

Serve accompanied by crudités or whole wheat bread croutons.

Sweet and sour onions

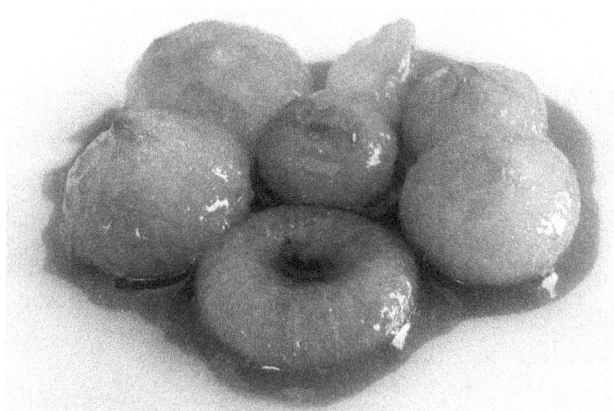

There should be some cooking liquid left, the "sauce", but if it is too much you can evaporate it by cooking uncovered for a few minutes.

Ingredients

- ~ 600 g of borettane onions
- ~ 3 tablespoons of extra virgin olive oil
- ~ 2 tablespoons of tamari or shoyu (soy sauce)
- ~ 1 tablespoon of rice acidulate
- ~ 2 tablespoons of rice malt
- ~ 1 pinch of whole sea salt

Instructions

Sauté the onions in a pan with the oil, salt and a little water for 5 minutes. Add a little more water and cook covered for 30 minutes. Check occasionally that there is always a little liquid in the bottom of the pan so that it doesn't burn.

Add the shoyu and cook for another 10-15 minutes, or until the onions are cooked through. At the end of the cooking time, add the malt and vinegar, stir and cook for another 1 minute and it's ready.

Baked grapes

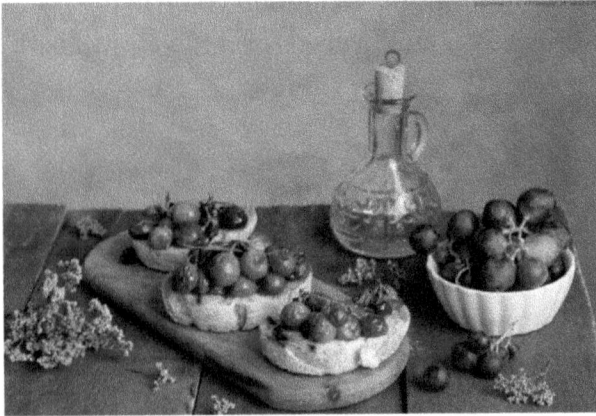

Ingredients for the baked grapes:

- ~ 500 g black table grapes
- ~ 2 tablespoons of extra virgin olive oil
- ~ 4-5 sprigs of thyme
- ~ salt

For the chapati:

- ~ 100 g whole wheat flour from ancient grains
- ~ 1 level teaspoon of whole sea salt
- ~ water

Instructions

Mix the flour and salt with enough water to knead and get an elastic ball. Let it rest covered with a damp cloth in a place protected from drafts, for 30 minutes.

Separate the berries from the stalks and cut about one third in half. The others remain whole. Transfer all the berries, both whole and halved, to a bowl and season with the oil, a pinch of salt and the thyme leaves. Mix well and transfer to a baking sheet lined with parchment paper. Bake at 200° for 15-20 minutes. When some berries begin to crack, the grapes are ready.

After the resting time, divide the dough into two balls and roll them out with a rolling pin forming two thin disks about 3 mm thick.

Leave to rest covered with a damp cloth for another 30 minutes.

Heat a non-stick frying pan or crêpes pan well and cook the disks one at a time on both sides, pressing lightly with a wooden spoon. They should puff up a little.

Keep them warm covered with a dry dish towel until you bring them to the table whole or cut into triangles accompanied by baked grapes and their sauce. You can use this particular recipe as an appetizer, snack or dessert.

Zucchini fritters with chickpea flour batter

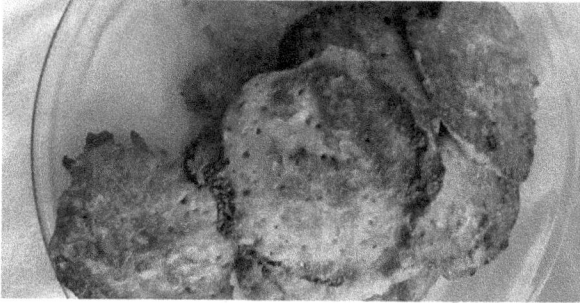

Fry the fritters on both sides and pat dry with some paper towels to remove excess oil.

A sprinkling of sweet paprika and they are ready. They are delicious hot, but also at room temperature.

Ingredients

~ 80 g of chickpea flour
~ 100 ml of water
~ 2 small or 1 large zucchini
~ 2 tablespoons of extra virgin olive oil
~ 1 level teaspoon of salt
~ 10 basil leaves
~ sweet paprika
~ oil for frying (the best is evo, if possible)

Instructions

Mix the chickpea flour with water and let it sit for 1 hour.

If you already have zucchini ready like I had, or other leftover vegetables, you can use those, otherwise you can grate the zucchini.

Add the salt to the chickpea batter and mix well, then add the zucchini, the 2 tablespoons of oil, the basil and mix well again.

Heat the oil in a frying pan and when hot pour in the batter by spoonfuls.

First Courses

Venus rice fantasy of spices

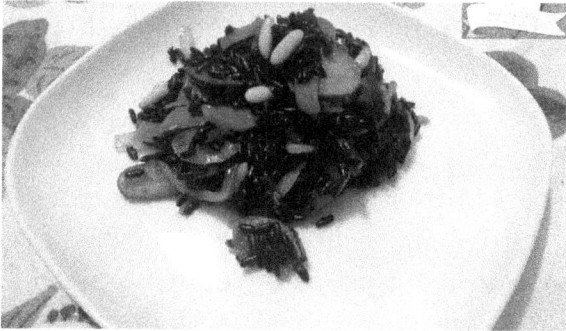

Ingredients for 2-3 people:

~ 200 g Venus rice
~ 150 g of cooked chickpeas
~ 2 carrots
~ 1 red onion
~ 1 garlic clove
~ the green part of 1 spring onion
~ a handful of sprouts
~ the juice of half a lime or lemon
~ the peel of half a lime or lemon
~ 2 tablespoons of extra virgin olive oil
~ 1 tablespoon of soy sauce
~ ½ teaspoon of curry
~ 1 pinch of tandoori (optional)
~ 1 pinch of garam masala (optional)
~ whole sea salt

Instructions

Wash the Venus rice and let it soak 6-8 hours. Soaking is not essential, so if you don't have time to soak it, cook it directly after washing it, as I did in this case, precisely because I didn't have time for soaking.

Cook the rice in a pressure cooker with 2x the amount of water and a pinch of salt, for about 20-25 minutes.

I measured 1 1/2 cups of rice, so I added 3 generous cups of water.

When cooked, turn off the heat and let rest, covered.

Meanwhile, thinly slice the onion and peel the garlic. Transfer them to a pan to brown with the oil, a pinch of salt, curry powder, tandoori and garam masala.

Stir often so the spices don't burn.

Cut the carrots into matchsticks or strips and add them to the pan. Add a splash of water and cover to cook 5 minutes.

Add the cooked chickpeas, the thinly sliced green part of the spring onion and the soy sauce and cook for a few more minutes, stirring.

Using a potato peeler, peel part of the lime or lemon and cut some slices of peel into strips.

At the end of cooking, add the peel, the juice of half a lime or lemon and the sprouts to the pan. If you use lemon instead of lime, halve the amount of juice.

Stir well and serve with Venus rice.

Venus rice with baked pumpkin and pistachio pesto

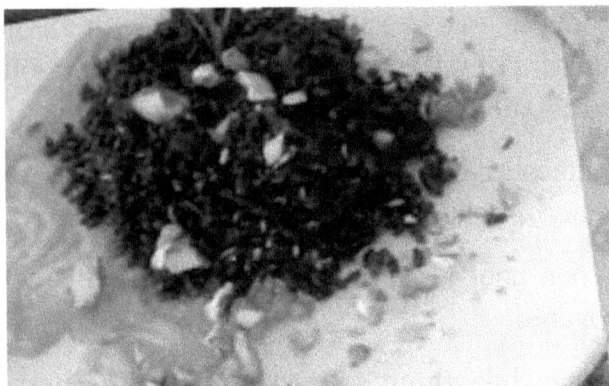

Ingredients for 2 people:

~ 150 g Venus rice
~ 1 small pumpkin (I used Hokkaido green pumpkin)
~ 1 teaspoon of mustard
~ ½ teaspoon umeboshi puree
~ 1 teaspoon rice acidulate or apple cider vinegar
~ 1 teaspoon ginger juice
~ chives
~ 2-3 mint leaves
~ 3-4 teaspoons of pistachio pesto
~ extra virgin olive oil
~ tamari

Instructions

Wash the Venus rice and boil it with twice the volume of water and a pinch of salt for about 20 minutes.

Wash the pumpkin well before opening it, using a small coconut brush to clean the skin, which can be eaten if it is thin.

Cut it into 4 and slice it. Clean the seeds from each slice and arrange the slices on a greased or lined baking sheet.

Mix 4-5 tablespoons of oil with 1 tablespoon of shoyu or tamari and brush the pumpkin slices with this mixture on both sides. Bake at 200° for 15-20 minutes, until the squash is well cooked.

Prepare the rice dressing by mixing the mustard, umeboshi puree, vinegar, ginger juice and 2 teaspoons of pistachio pesto. Cut some chive stems into small cylinders and chop 2-3 mint leaves.

Season the cooked rice with this dressing, the chives and mint.

Servi accompagnando con la zucca al forno e un po' di pesto al pistacchio.

Brown rice with pumpkin

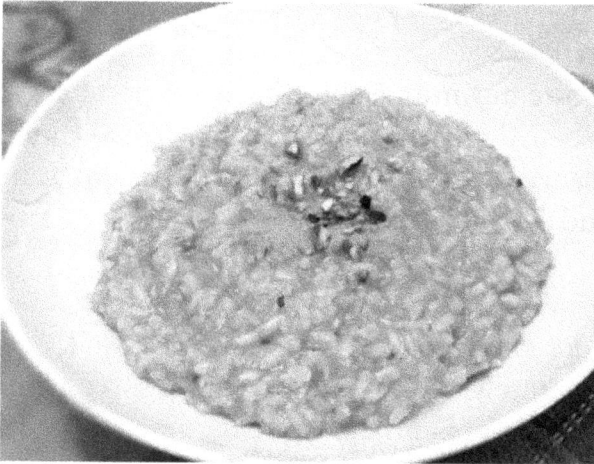

Ingredients

~ 300 g of brown rice
~ 1 litre of water (about)
~ 400 g of cleaned pumpkin cut into cubes
~ 1 large onion (about 250 g)
~ 3 tablespoons extra-virgin olive oil or sesame oil
~ 3-4 tablespoons unsweetened soy or oat cream
~ a pinch of whole sea salt
~ 1 pinch of black pepper (optional)
~ 3 pinches of turmeric
~ chopped parsley
~ tamari

Instructions

Wash the rice and put it in a pot with the water, salt, chopped onion and half of the pumpkin cut into cubes that will break up during cooking creating a cream.

Bring to the boil, then lower the heat and cook with the lid on, leaving a small gap, for about 20-30 minutes. At this point add the rest of the diced pumpkin, oil, turmeric and pepper. Cook for another 10-15 minutes, but taste the rice so as not to scald it. If you need to cook longer, but the water has already absorbed, you can add some, preferably hot.

A few minutes from the end of cooking, add the cream and stir well to blend.

Taste and if necessary add a little tamari or shoyu.

Finally, add chopped parsley and serve.

Brown rice with spring onions and sautéed tempeh

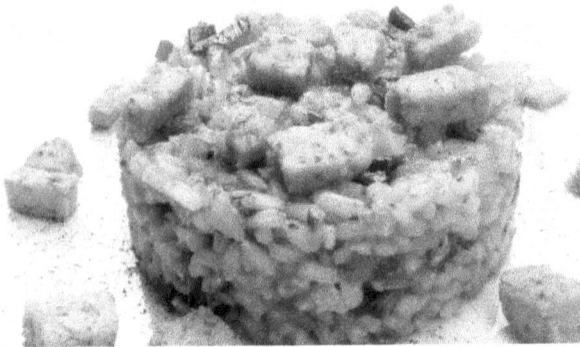

Ingredients

- ~ 300 g of cooked brown rice
- ~ 150 g of natural tempeh
- ~ 2 spring onions
- ~ 2 tablespoons of tamari
- ~ 1 teaspoon rice vinegar (or apple vinegar)
- ~ whole sea salt
- ~ extra virgin olive oil or sesame oil
- ~ ½ teaspoon of curry
- ~ sweet paprika

Instructions

Dice the tempeh and brown it in a pan with 2 tablespoons of oil, the curry powder and a pinch of salt. Move it often with a spoon because it tends to stick. Brown it well for a few minutes and at the end add the rice vinegar. If you use apple vinegar, reduce the quantity because it is stronger.

Cut the spring onion, separating the green part, which you will keep aside. Finely slice the white part and sauté it in a pan (a different one from the one with the tempeh) with a tablespoon of oil and a pinch of salt.

In the meantime, slice the green part as well. When the spring onion in the pan is almost ready, add the green part and the soy sauce and cook for 1 minute.

Add the cooked rice and mix well. Add separately browned tempeh and serve with a sprinkle of paprika.

Pumpkin Basmati Risotto

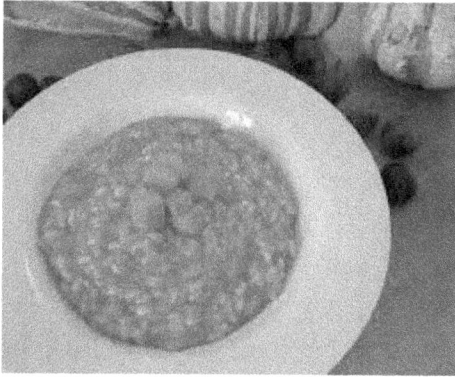

Ingredients for about 2 people

- ~ 150 g brown basmati rice
- ~ 200 g of cleaned pumpkin
- ~ 1 onion
- ~ 2 tablespoon oil
- ~ vegetable broth
- ~ 1 pinch of whole sea salt
- ~ cream of balsamic or apple vinegar (optional)

Instructions

Thinly slice the onion and sauté in a pan with the oil, salt and a little water until golden brown. Add the washed basmati rice and let it toast, stirring for a couple of minutes.

Add the pumpkin cut into small cubes and 2-3 ladles of hot stock. Bring to the boil and begin the typical risotto cooking process, which calls for gradually adding broth during cooking when the rice gets too dry. Cook for about 20 minutes, but taste the rice after 15 minutes.

Asparagus rice with a creamy sauce

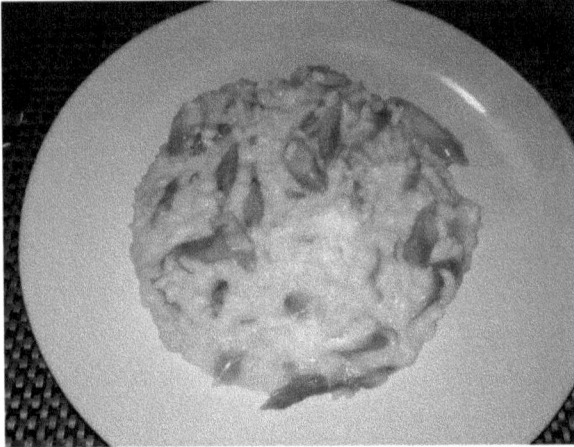

Ingredients

- ~ 500 g of asparagus
- ~ ½ chopped onion
- ~ 1 glass of semi-integral rice
- ~ white wine (optional)
- ~ vegetable broth
- ~ 1 tablespoon tamari or shoyu (soy sauce)
- ~ extra virgin olive oil

Instructions

Clean the asparagus and go through the stalks with a potato peeler. Cut off the hardest part of the stalks and set aside. Cut the asparagus into rounds, leaving the tips whole.

Fry the onion with a pinch of salt, add the asparagus slices, leaving the tips aside. Add the rice and toast it for a few minutes.

Deglaze with a little white wine. Add some broth and let it cook. Semi-whole rice cooks in about 20 minutes.

Boil in boiling salted water the hard stalks set aside and once cooked, blend them with a little oil and tamari, to obtain a cream.

Continue cooking the rice, adding broth as needed. After about 15 minutes of cooking, add the asparagus tips and continue cooking another 5-10 minutes.

Adjust the salt. As soon as the rice is cooked, add the blended stalks sauce to cream the rice.

Spiced brown basmati rice with green beans

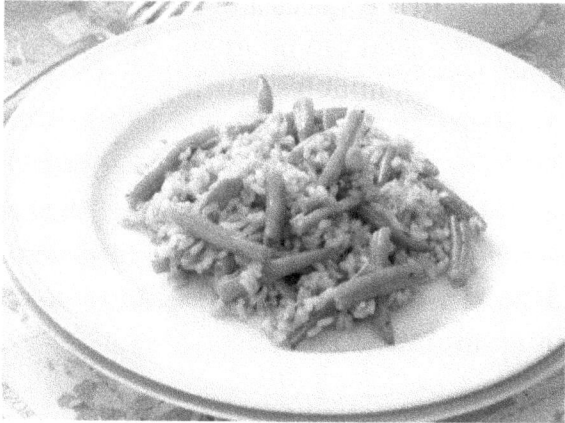

Ingredients for about 2 people:

~ 150 g brown basmati rice

~ 200 g of green beans

~ various herbs to taste (basil, thyme, etc.)

~ 1 teaspoon of sweet curry

~ 1 pinch of cumin

~ 1 tablespoon umeboshi acidulate (optional)

~ 1 garlic clove

~ 2 tablespoons extra virgin olive oil

~ 1 pinch of whole sea salt

Instructions

Wash the rice and let it soak a few hours. Discard the soaking water and boil it with twice the volume of water and a pinch of salt for 10-15 minutes, partially covered. At the end of the cooking time, when the water has been absorbed, turn off the heat and let it rest, covered, for 10 minutes.

While the rice is cooking, sauté the green beans cut into small cylinders in a pan with oil, garlic and a pinch of salt for a few minutes. Add a little water and leave to cook, covered, for 10 minutes. When cooked, remove the garlic.

Transfer the rice to a pan brushed with oil and add the spices, cumin and curry. Sauté the rice for 1 minute, stirring well. Turn off the heat and add the umeboshi acidulate.

You can serve the rice accompanied by the green beans, or mix them together, or plate as in the photo, using a pastry cup or mold to shape the rice and cover with the green beans.

Brown basmati rice with pumpkin and chickpeas

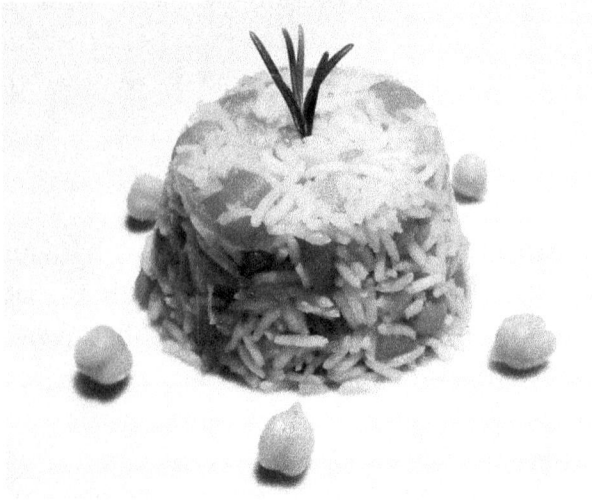

Dice the pumpkin and keep it aside. Thinly slice the onion and garlic and brown them in a pan with oil and a little water for a few minutes. Add the spices and let them toast for 1-2 minutes. Add the pumpkin and chickpeas and sauté for 5 minutes, stirring well.

Add ½ cup of water and let it stew, covered, for 15-20 minutes. When pumpkin is cooked add tamari or shoyu and rice and cook for another minute stirring.

Ingredients

- ~ 150 g of brown basmati rice
- ~ 1 onion
- ~ 1 garlic clove (optional)
- ~ 300 g of cleaned pumpkin
- ~ 150 g boiled chickpeas
- ~ 1 teaspoon of turmeric (or more, to taste)
- ~ 1 teaspoon of curry powder (or more, to taste)
- ~ 1 teaspoon of sweet paprika (or more, to taste)
- ~ 2 tablespoons extra-virgin olive oil
- ~ 2 tablespoons tamari or shoyu (soy sauce)

Instructions

Wash the rice and boil it with twice the volume of water and a pinch of salt, partially covered for about 20 minutes. When the rice is cooked, turn off the heat and let it rest, covered.

Brown rice with green beans and raisins

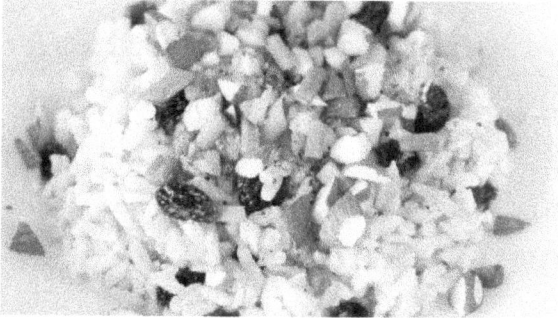

In the meantime, soak the raisins for a few minutes and when they are ready, squeeze them and transfer them to the pan.

When green beans are ready add boiled rice, stir and serve hot or at room temperature, garnishing with a mint leaf or gomasio.

Ingredients

- ~ 150 g brown rice
- ~ 2-3 handfuls of green beans
- ~ 2 tablespoons of raisins
- ~ 1 leek
- ~ 2 tablespoons extra virgin olive oil
- ~ 2 tablespoons of tamari
- ~ whole sea salt

Instructions

Soak the rice overnight or for a day, then throw out the water and cook it with twice the volume of water and a pinch of salt for about 20-25 minutes, partially covered. When cooked, let it rest covered for 10 minutes.

Slice the leek and fry it in a pan with oil, a pinch of salt and a little water. If you want, you can do this without oil, just with salt and water.

Meanwhile, cut the green beans into small cylinders and add them to the pan. Season with shoyu or tamari and, if necessary, add a little water and cook for about 10 minutes.

Whole wheat basmati rice with asparagus seitan ragout

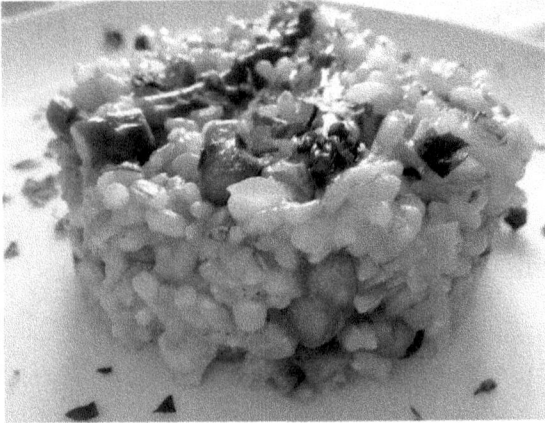

Ingredients

- ~ 1 cup of brown basmati rice (if soaked a few hours is better)
- ~ 100 g of seitan
- ~ 1 tablespoon extra virgin olive oil
- ~ 1 pinch of whole sea salt
- ~ 1 bay leaf
- ~ 1 sprig of rosemary
- ~ 3 leaves of sage
- ~ 1 onion
- ~ 400 g of asparagus

Instructions

Wash the rice well and cook it with two generous cups of water and 1 pinch of salt for about 20 minutes.

Boil the asparagus in boiling salted water.

Chop the onion thinly and brown it in a pan with oil and a pinch of salt. Chop the seitan finely and add it to the pan. Chop the rosemary and sage and transfer them to the pan. Add the bay leaf as well.

If necessary, add a little water and cook for 10 minutes.

In the meantime, cut off the asparagus tips and set them aside. Blend the stalks and pass the mixture through a vegetable mill to remove the fibrous part and obtain a puree.

Put the puree in the pan, stir and turn off. Add the boiled rice and stir gently.

Brown basmati rice with broccoli

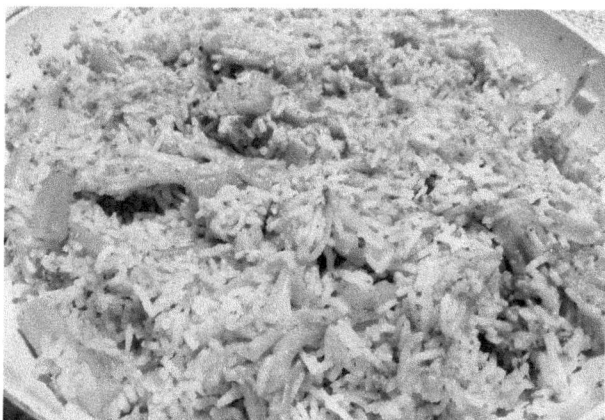

Ingredients

~ 1 cup brown basmati rice
~ 1-2 broccoli (depending on size) with stem and leaves (if any)
~ 1 garlic clove
~ 3 tablespoons extra virgin olive oil
~ 3 tablespoons of tamari or shoyu (soy sauce)
~ 2 tablespoons desalted capers
~ 1 teaspoon of mustard
~ 1/2 teaspoon of balsamic vinegar
~ 2 teaspoons of umeboshi acidulate

Instructions

Wash and boil rice with 2 parts water and a pinch of salt for 20 minutes, partially covered. When cooked, turn off the heat and let rest for 10 minutes.

In the meantime, clean the broccoli stalk and slice it into very thin julienne strips and season with the balsamic vinegar and umeboshi acidulate, leaving it to marinate.

Thinly slice the garlic and fry it in a pan with 2 tablespoons of oil. Add the broccoli florets, sauté for 2 minutes and then stew covered for 5 minutes.

Add a little water if necessary. When cooked, add 2 tablespoons of tamari and cook for a few more minutes.

If the broccoli still has its leaves, you can cut them into strips and add them to the pan, cooking for 2 minutes. They are delicious!

Blend half of the broccoli in the pan with 1 tablespoon of oil, 1 of tamari, the capers, mustard and a little water to make a smooth, creamy mixture. Mix the rice with the other half of the broccoli.

Arrange the rice in the center of the plate and decorate with the broccoli sauce. Arrange a few julienne of marinated broccoli stalks on top of the rice.

Obviously it is not essential to compose the dish in this way; if you are in a hurry you can simply mix the rice with the broccoli, the sauce and arrange the julienne on top.

Brown rice with cauliflower and prunes

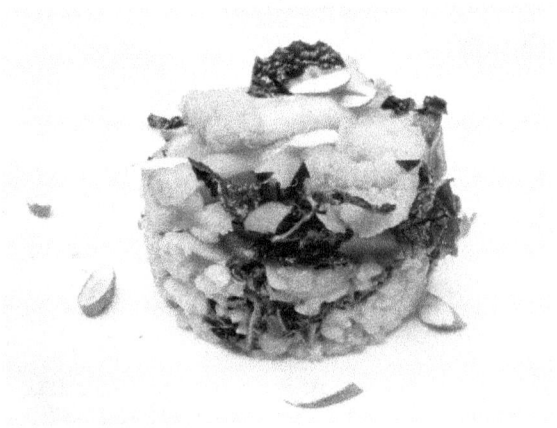

Now combine all the ingredients in a pan: the rice, cauliflower florets, plums and chives.

If you have already boiled rice and cauliflower it's really easy, just chop the plums and chives!

Add the oil and tamari (or shoyu) and sauté for a couple of minutes.

Serve with a sprinkle of gomasio.

Ingredients

- ~ 150 g of brown rice
- ~ 10-12 prunes
- ~ 1/2 small cauliflower (or more, as desired)
- ~ 1 tablespoon of extra virgin olive oil
- ~ 2 tablespoons of tamari
- ~ chives (or other flavourings to taste)
- ~ gomasio

Instructions

After soaking the rice for about 8 hours, boil it with twice as much water and a pinch of salt, for about 20-30 minutes, covered.

Steam the cauliflower or boil it in boiling salted water.

Cut the plums into small pieces and chop the chives.

Rosemary buckwheat with caramelized pumpkin

Mix the buckwheat with the sour cream and chopped rosemary.

You can serve separately as I did, or mix the squash with the buckwheat.

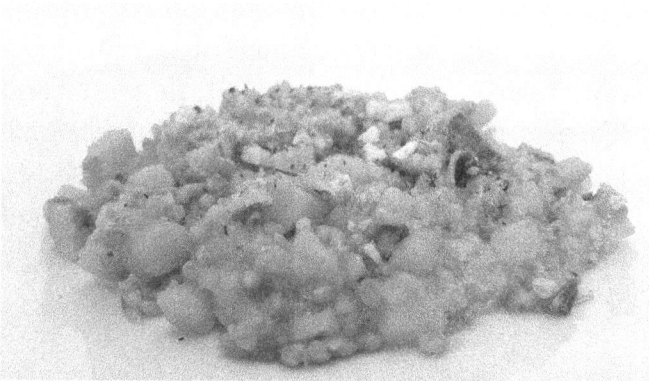

Ingredients

- ~ 1 cup of hulled buckwheat (about 150 g)
- ~ 500 g of cleaned pumpkin
- ~ 2 tablespoons of extra virgin olive oil
- ~ 2 tablespoons of shoyu or tamari (soy sauce)
- ~ 2 tablespoons of rice malt
- ~ 1 teaspoon umeboshi acidulate
- ~ 1 sprig of rosemary

Instructions

Wash the buckwheat well and boil it with a little more than twice as much water and a pinch of salt for about 15 minutes, covered, leaving only a small gap for the steam to pass through. At the end of cooking turn off the flame and leave it covered to rest for 10 minutes.

In the meantime, cut the pumpkin into small cubes and brown it in a pan with oil for a few minutes. Add the tamari and malt and cook, stirring until soft.

Rice and Beans

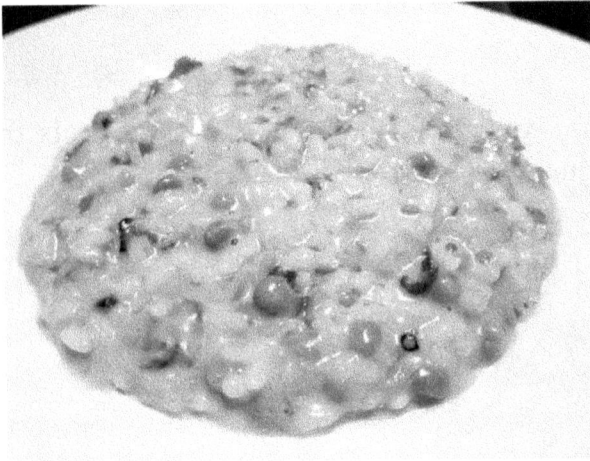

Ingredients

- ~ 200 g of semi-integral rice
- ~ 200 g dry split peas (soaked for a few hours)
- ~ 1 onion
- ~ 1 carrot
- ~ 1 litre of vegetable stock (1 onion, 1 carrot, 1 celery stalk, 1 piece of kombu)
- ~ parsley
- ~ 3 cm of kombu seaweed
- ~ whole sea salt
- ~ 2 tablespoons extra virgin olive oil

Instructions

After soaking the peas, change the water and cook them with the kombu seaweed for 30-45 minutes or until soft.

In the meantime, prepare the broth by putting in a pot 1 litre of water with 1 peeled onion cut in half, 1 carrot, 1 stalk of celery and 1 piece of kombu.

Bring to a boil and cook for 20-30 minutes.

Chop the onion, grate the carrot and sauté in a pan with the oil and a pinch of salt for a few minutes. If necessary, add a little water and leave to stew, covered, for 20 minutes. This long and unusual cooking time allows you to "extract" the sweet flavor of the carrot and onion.

Add the rice and let it toast for a few minutes while stirring, then add 2-3 ladles of broth, a good pinch of salt, bring to a boil and start calculating about 20 minutes of cooking time. Lower the heat and add more broth as the stock dries. The last 10 minutes of cooking add the boiled peas.

At the end of the cooking time add the parsley and, if necessary, add salt to taste.

Rice noodles with vegetables

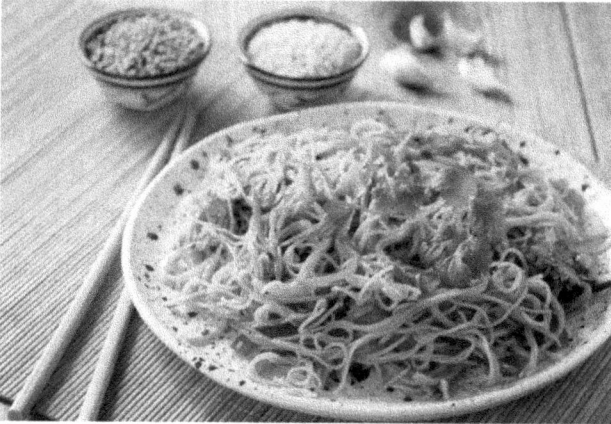

Cook about 5 minutes, stirring often. When the vegetables are al dente, add the sprouts and sauté for another 1 minute. Turn off the heat and add the ginger and lemon juice and chives.

Some people boil the noodles in boiling salted water for 5-6 minutes and some people let them soak in boiling water for 10 minutes. Drain the noodles and transfer them to the pan with the vegetables.

Rice noodles tend to stick together even if they are al dente. Use two forks or a fork and tongs to untangle them.

Or you can run them under water quickly after they are cooked.

Immediately transfer them to the pan with the vegetables, mix well and serve decorating to taste with chives, gomasio, etc..

Ingredients for 2-3 people:

~ 250 g brown rice noodles
~ 1 piece of leek (about 10 cm)
~ 1 piece of daikon or 4-5 radishes
~ 2 carrots
~ 4 cabbage leaves
~ 2 handfuls of sprouts
~ 2 tablespoons of tamari
~ 1 pinch of curry powder
~ 1 tablespoon ginger juice
~ 1 tablespoon lemon juice
~ 2 tablespoons extra virgin olive oil or sesame oil
~ whole sea salt
~ chives

Instructions

Cut the leek and cabbage into strips and the carrot and daikon into thin sticks or matchsticks. Sauté the carrots and daikon in a pan with the oil, 1 pinch of salt and curry powder for a few minutes, then add the leek, cabbage and soy sauce.

Tofu with béchamel sauce and caramelized onions

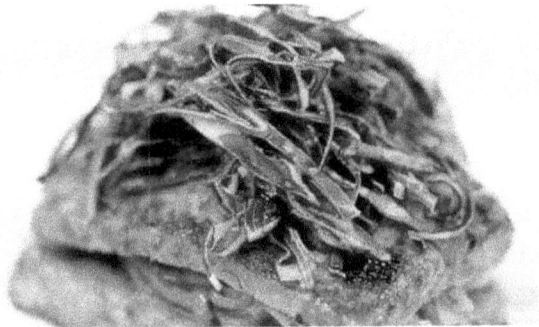

Ingredients for the malfatti:

~ 2 heads of chard or 4 heads of spinach
~ 100 g of natural tofu
~ chopped mixed herbs (sage, thyme, etc.)
~ 5 tablespoons of flour type 1 or type 2
~ whole sea salt

For the caramelized onions

~ 1 red onion
~ 1 tablespoon of rice malt
~ 1 tablespoon tamari or shoyu (soy sauce)
~ 1 tablespoon extra virgin olive oil
~ gomasio to taste

For the béchamel

~ 250 g unsweetened soy or oat milk
~ 1 tablespoon and a half of semi-wholemeal flour type 1 or type 2
~ 1/2 teaspoon integral sea salt
~ evo oil
~ nutmeg

Instructions

Boil the chard and tofu in plenty of boiling salted water. Prepare the chopped herbs with rosemary, sage, thyme, mint, chives, or others to taste. Drain the chard without draining the water and leave to cool.

In the meantime, slice the onions thinly and fry them in a pan with 1 tablespoon of oil for 1-2 minutes, then add the malt and tamari and let them cook and caramelize 5-10 minutes.

Put the soy milk on the stove with half a teaspoon of salt and a little nutmeg. In the meantime, mix the flour with a little corn oil, just enough to make a fairly liquid batter. Bring the milk to a boil and pour in the batter, stirring with a whisk. Cook 2-3 minutes stirring and when the béchamel has thickened well, turn off the heat.

Squeeze the chard very well and blend with the tofu and chopped herbs. Transfer the mixture to a bowl, add 5 tablespoons of flour and a pinch of salt. Mix well, taste and adjust salt if necessary. Shape the "malfatti" into small balls or cylinders. Bring the water in which you boiled the chard and tofu back to the boil and cook the malfatti for a few minutes. When they tend to come to the surface, they are ready. Transfer them to the pan with the béchamel sauce and stir gently.

Accompany the malfatti with béchamel sauce with the caramelized onions and a sprinkling of gomasio.

Couscous dumplings

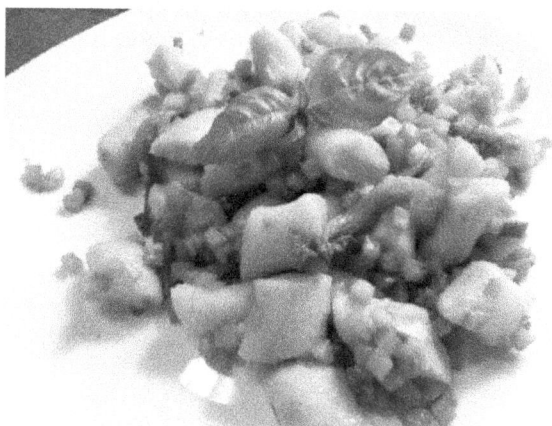

Ingredients for 3-4 people:

For the gnocchi

~ 200-250 g wholemeal couscous (corn or rice for those with gluten intolerance)
~ 500 ml water
~ 1 pinch of whole sea salt
~ For the dressing
~ 2 large whole leeks
~ 2 small carrots
~ 2 tablespoons of extra virgin olive oil
~ 2 tablespoons shoyu or a pinch of salt

Instructions

Bring water to a boil with a pinch of salt. When it boils, pour in the cous cous, stir and cook for 2 minutes. Turn off and stir well for a few minutes, breaking up the cous cous. Try to compact it well and let it rest covered for 10 minutes.

Depending on the type of cous cous used (wheat, kamut, spelt, corn, etc..) may vary the amount of water needed. Try with the one of the recipe and eventually the next time adjust the quantity according to the cous cous you are

using. If the first time it is not the perfect amount, do not worry, at most it will remain a bit hard, but it is still good. If it is too soft, add some flour.

While the cous cous is resting, prepare the dressing.

Slice the leeks thinly and brown them in a pan with oil and a pinch of salt or shoyu. In the meantime grate the carrots and add them to the pan. If necessary, add a little water and leave to stew, covered, for 10 minutes.

In the meantime the couscous will have cooled down. Turn it out onto a work surface and knead it with your hands until the grains of the cous cous are no longer felt and a smooth dough forms.

Divide the dough to form cylinders 1- 1.5 cm in diameter. Cut small dumplings, about 1 inch in size, and flour them.

If the leeks and carrots didn't flake enough during cooking, you can blend to make the topping creamier. I didn't blend.

Transfer the gnocchi to the pan with the vegetables, add a little water and let them cook a few minutes, stirring gently. It is not necessary to cook them in water because the cous cous is already cooked.

Serve with a sprinkling of gomasio.

Fusilli with cream of zucchini

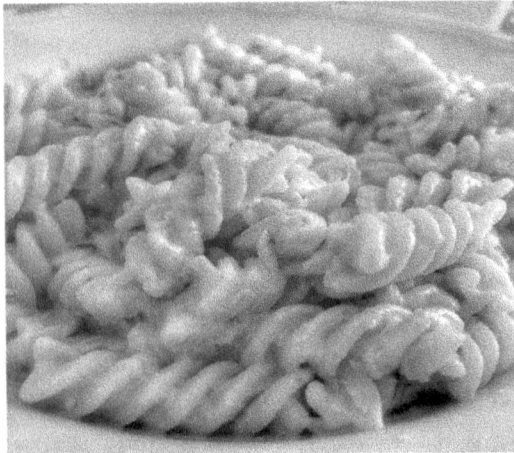

A sprinkling of gomasio and it's ready. You can enjoy this pasta hot or fresh as a pasta salad.

Ingredients for 2 people:

- ~ 200 g of whole wheat pasta made of spelt or ancient grains
- ~ 4 zucchini
- ~ 1 shallot
- ~ 1 pinch of whole sea salt
- ~ 1-2 tablespoons of shoyu (soy sauce)
- ~ 3-4 tablespoons of olives
- ~ 3-4 basil leaves
- ~ 2-3 mint leaves
- ~ 2 tablespoons of extra virgin olive oil

Instructions

Thinly slice the shallot and brown it in a pan with oil, salt and a little water. Meanwhile, cut the zucchini into cubes. When shallot is wilted, add zucchini and shoyu and cook for about 5 minutes until zucchini is soft. Meanwhile, cook the pasta.

Remove about half of the zucchini from the pan and blend with the basil and mint. Add a little water if needed. Transfer back to the pan and add the olives and drained pasta.

Whole wheat fusilli with broccoli and prunes

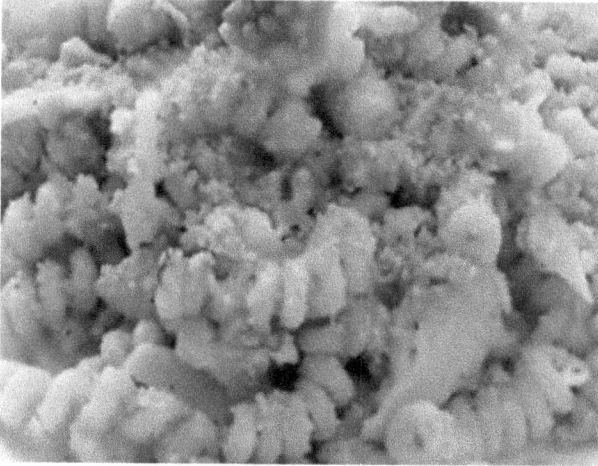

Ingredients

- ~ 100 g of whole wheat pasta made from ancient grains or spelt
- ~ a little boiled broccoli (I know, it's not very professional "a little", but I was in a hurry!)
- ~ a handful of prunes
- ~ tamari or shoyu (soy sauce)
- ~ gomasio

Instructions

Boil the fusilli. Meanwhile, quickly sauté the chopped broccoli in a skillet. If you like you can add a clove of garlic. Add chopped plums and season with tamari or shoyu. Add the fusilli, stir-fry for 1 minute and serve with a sprinkling of gomasio.

Enjoy!

Leek cannelloni stuffed with tofu and walnuts

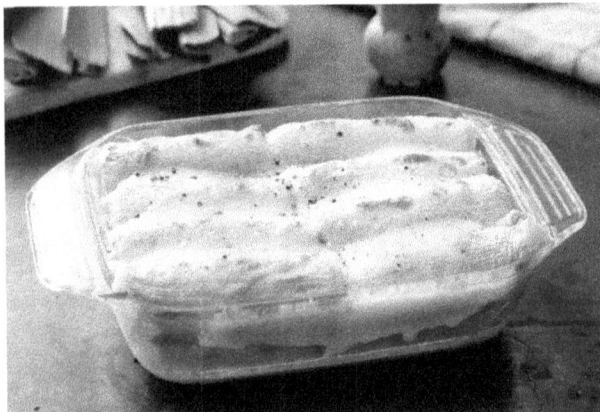

Ingredients

- ~ 1 rather large leek
- ~ 100 g of natural tofu
- ~ 50 g of walnut kernels
- ~ 1 small teaspoon of turmeric
- ~ ½ teaspoon sweet curry
- ~ 2 tablespoons tamari
- ~ 2 tablespoons extra virgin olive oil
- ~ 1 teaspoon umeboshi acidulate

For the reduction:

- ~ 3 tablespoons tamari
- ~ 1 teaspoon rice vinegar
- ~ 2 tablespoons clear apple juice

Instructions

Cut off the end of the leek to remove the root. Also cut off the part where the tougher leaves begin and keep it aside. You will have obtained a cylinder. Cut along the top of the leek to open it up a bit and remove the first outer leaf, which should be discarded.

Now cut cylinders about 2 inches long. Separate the leaves to get 8-10 small cylinders open on one side and set them aside. Wash them under water if necessary.

Clean the rest of the leek, cut it into rounds and transfer them to a pan with 2 tablespoons of oil, a little water, turmeric and curry. Sauté for a few minutes, then add the tamari and let it stew for 5 minutes.

Blend the tofu with the stewed leeks and umeboshi acidulate. Chop up half the walnuts and add them to the tofu-leek mixture. Stuff the leek cylinders with the mixture and brush with oil. Bake at 350°F for 15-20 minutes.

Meanwhile, reduce leftover walnuts to flour and prepare soy sauce reduction.

Put the shoyu, vinegar and apple juice in a pan and cook over high heat, stirring occasionally, for a few minutes, until the liquid has dried and thickened.

Serve the leek cannelloni sprinkled with the walnut flour and a few drops of shoyu reduction.

Panzerotti stuffed with chard and tofu

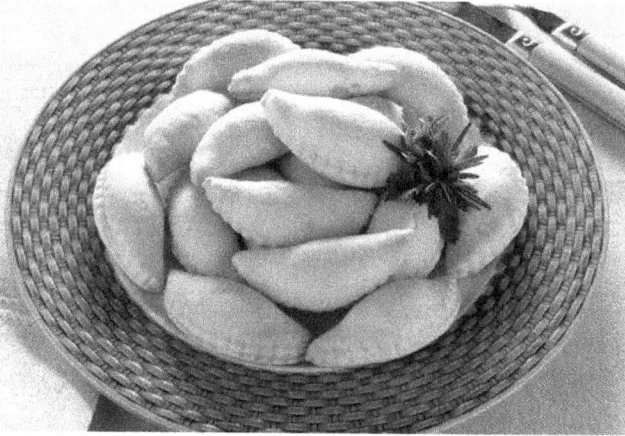

Ingredients for about 15 panzerotti

For the dough:

- ~ 120 g whole wheat flour
- ~ 30 g of corn flour
- ~ 50 g of semi-whole wheat flour
- ~ 2 tablespoons of extra virgin olive oil
- ~ 1 pinch of integral sea salt
- ~ ½ teaspoon of natural yeast (optional)
- ~ water

For the filling

- ~ 200 g chard (green part only) or spinach
- ~ 1 garlic clove
- ~ 80 g of tofu
- ~ 2 tablespoons of extra virgin olive oil
- ~ nutmeg
- ~ 1 tablespoon of white miso (or half a tablespoon of classic miso)
- ~ 1 teaspoon of tahini
- ~ thyme
- ~ sage
- ~ salt or soy sauce

Instructions

Prepare the dough by mixing the different flours, yeast, salt and oil. Add a little water to mix and get a fairly soft dough, to be placed in the refrigerator about 30 minutes wrapped in plastic wrap.

Meanwhile prepare the filling. Boil the chard and tofu in boiling salted water (in the same pot). When beets are tender, drain and squeeze well. Set the tofu aside. On a cutting board, chop the chard coarsely with a knife. Put them in a frying pan with oil and chopped garlic, chopped sage and thyme. Blend the tofu, but briefly, so as not to make it too smooth, or chop it with a knife.

Mix the miso with the tahin and a little water to make a cream.

Combine the chard, tofu, tahini and miso cream and nutmeg in a bowl. Taste and add soy sauce or salt if necessary.

Now roll out the dough very thin. Cut discs using a pastry cutter or cup. I used a 9 cm diameter pasta cup.

On each disc place a little bit of filling, only one half of the disc, so you can fold the dough in half obtaining a half moon. Close the panzerotto by pressing the edge with your fingers.

Place the panzerotti on a baking sheet with baking paper and brush them with a little oil. I prepared a mixture of oil, tamari and a pinch of turmeric, but just a little oil is fine too.

After brushing them on, I sprinkled poppy seeds for garnish. You can use sesame seeds as well.

Bake at 170° for 30-40 minutes. After about 20 minutes it's best to flip them.

Asparagus crepes with white miso sauce

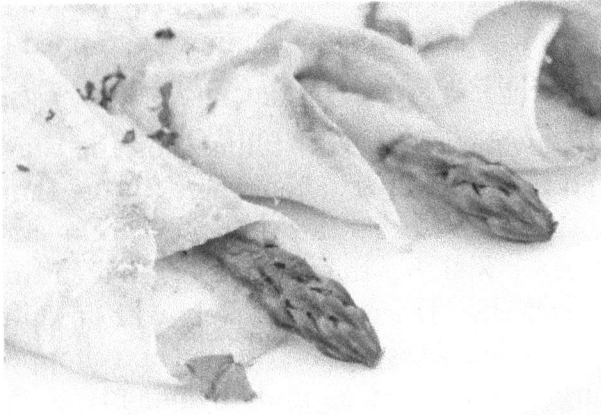

Ingredients for 4 crepes of 15 cm in diameter

- ~ 400 g of semi-whole wheat flour type 1 or type 2
- ~ 50 g of corn flour
- ~ ½ teaspoon of integral sea salt
- ~ 300-350 ml water
- ~ 500 g of asparagus
- ~ For the sauce
- ~ 2 tablespoons clear tahin
- ~ 1 tablespoon shiro miso
- ~ water

Instructions

Remove the end part of the stem of the asparagus (3-4 cm) and boil it in boiling salted water.

In the meantime, prepare the sauce by mixing the miso, tahin and enough water to make a smooth sauce. If you have never used tahini, you should know that it does not mix easily with liquids, so you need to mix it well.

Prepare the crepe batter by mixing the two flours with the salt and water a little at a time. Mix well with a whisk so that no lumps form.

Heat a small frying pan well, adding a little oil, about ½ teaspoon. I use a pan with a bottom of about 15 cm in diameter because it allows me to handle the crepes well, turning them without effort and without breaking them.

When the oil is hot pour a ladleful of the mixture, move the pan so that it is distributed all over the bottom and cook for about 1 minute. With a soft silicone scoop, shake the edges and shake the pan to dislodge the crepe from the bottom. Use the paddle if necessary, but if you've put enough oil in, it's not necessary. Flip the crepe using the paddle or "sauté" it.

Cook the other side well and set aside. Add more oil to the pan and make another crepe and so on until you have made 4.

Drain the asparagus and assemble the crepes: put in each crepe about 2 tablespoons of sauce, add 3-4 asparagus and close it. Prepare the others and, if necessary, put them in the oven to warm them up.

Crepes with leeks, shitake mushrooms and yogurt sauce

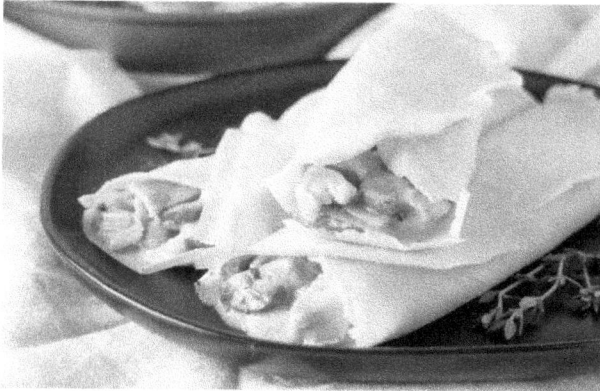

Ingredients for 3-4 crepes:

- ~ 100 g flour type 1 or type 2
- ~ 200 ml of water
- ~ 3 tablespoons of extra virgin olive oil
- ~ 1/2 teaspoon whole sea salt
- ~ 1/2 teaspoon of turmeric

For the filling

- ~ 2 leeks
- ~ 1 handful of dried shitake mushrooms (about 10 g)
- ~ 3 tablespoons extra virgin olive oil
- ~ 2 tablespoons tamari or shoyu

For the accompanying sauce

- ~ 100 g boiled chickpeas
- ~ 130 g of natural soy yogurt
- ~ 1 tablespoon extra virgin olive oil
- ~ 1 tablespoon of tamari
- ~ 1 tablespoon umeboshi acidulate

Instructions

Soak the mushrooms in warm water for about 10 minutes until soft. You can reuse the soaking water for a miso soup or soup. Shitakes are not earthy because they grow on trees.

While the mushrooms are soaking, slice the leek into thin rounds and sauté with the oil and a little water. Cut the mushrooms into thin slices and place them in the pan with the leeks. If they have been soaking long enough you can also use the stem, which will be soft. Let them brown 1-2 minutes, add a little water and let them stew covered for about 10 minutes.

In the meantime, prepare the sauce by blending the chickpeas with the oil, tamari, acidulates and a little yogurt. When you have obtained a homogeneous mixture, add the rest of the yogurt and blend again.

When the mushrooms are cooked, add the tamari or shoyu, cook for another minute and turn off the heat.

Mix the flour with the water, stirring with a whisk, and add the salt and turmeric. Prepare a large, flat non-stick frying pan by brushing it with oil. Put it on the stove to heat and when it is hot pouring a ladleful of batter, moving the pan so that it is distributed evenly, forming a thin layer. Cook about 1 minute, shaking the pan occasionally, then gently flip it over to cook on the other side. I use a paddle and my hands.

When it's ready, transfer it to a baking sheet lined with parchment paper and prepare the others, which you'll put in the pan as you go.

When you have all the crepes ready, you can stuff them. Arrange some mushrooms and leeks on half of the crepes and add a spoonful or two of yogurt sauce. Close the crepe and prepare the others in the same way. At the time of serving you can heat them in the oven and when they are in the garnish them with a little 'yogurt sauce and a sprinkling of nori seaweed flakes or poppy seeds or with a little 'gomasio.

Piadina with cream of onions and olives

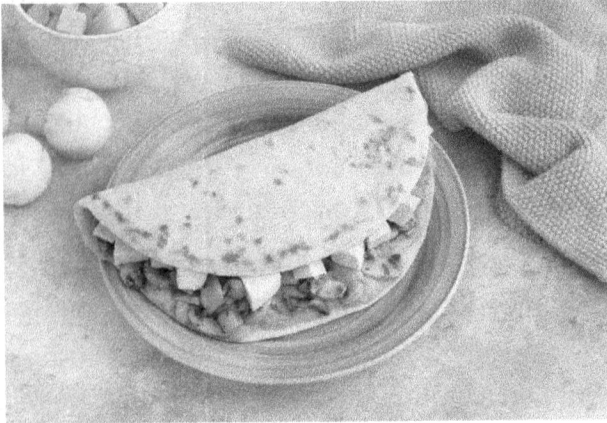

Ingredients

- ~ 3-4 piadine
- ~ 4 onions
- ~ 2 tablespoons of soy sauce
- ~ 1 tablespoon extra virgin olive oil
- ~ 1 pinch of salt
- ~ pitted black olives
- ~ oregano

Instructions

Peel the onions and cut them into slices. Transfer them to a pan with the oil, salt and a little water and stew until soft. In the last minutes of cooking, add the soy sauce and a little oregano.

Blend half of the onions to obtain a cream.

Prepare the piadina and stuff it with the onion cream, stewed sliced onions and olives.

Scrambled millet

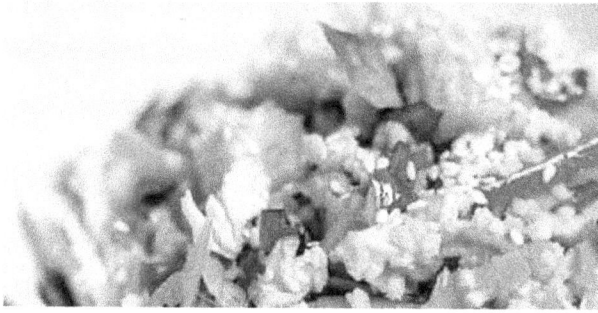

In a frying pan heat the oil and add the diced zucchini. Fry for a few minutes then add the diced tomato. Add a little water and cook for a few minutes. Add the tamari and cook until the vegetables are tender. Add boiled millet, chopped basil, stir and turn off. You can serve it hot, warm or room temperature.

Ingredients

- ~ 1 cup of husked millet
- ~ 2 ripe tomatoes
- ~ 1 zucchini
- ~ 1 tablespoon extra virgin olive oil
- ~ 2 tablespoons of tamari
- ~ basil
- ~ whole sea salt

Instructions

Wash the millet well and boil it with 2 and a half cups of water and a pinch of whole sea salt for about 15 minutes from boiling, covered, leaving only a small gap for the passage of steam. When cooked, turn off the heat and let rest, covered, for 10 minutes.

Depending on the brand, millet may have a cooking time ranging from 10 to 20 minutes, so experiment and find the right amount of water and cooking time for the millet you purchased. When the millet is almost ready you will see that it will have absorbed almost all the water and will be puffed up. At that point taste it and if it is not hard it is ready. Now turn it off and leave it covered for 10 minutes to finish absorbing the water.

Millet with almonds and arugula

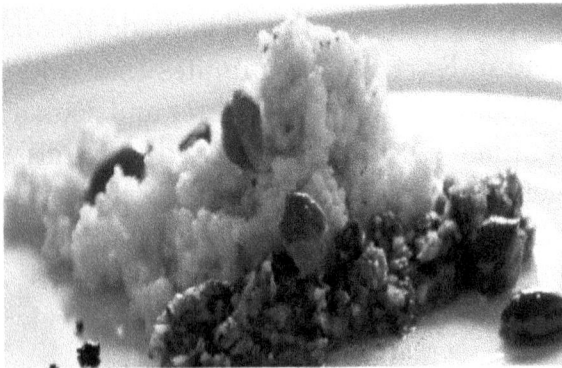

Ingredients

- ~ 150 g of husked millet
- ~ 80-100 g of almonds
- ~ 1 carrot
- ~ 1 small leek
- ~ 1 bunch of rocket
- ~ 2 tablespoons of tamari
- ~ 2 tablespoons of sesame seed oil or extra virgin olive oil

Instructions

As a first step toast the almonds in the oven for 10 minutes at 160 °. Do not let them out of your sight because they burn in an instant! Toasting the almonds makes them not only delicious, but also much more digestible.

Wash the millet well, drain and boil it with a little more than double the volume of water for 15 minutes with a pinch of salt, partially covered. Turn off the heat and leave to rest, covered. Slice the leek thinly and fry it in a pan with the oil and a little water.

Grate the carrot and add it to the pan. Add the tamari or shoyu and cook for a few more minutes. In the meantime, cut the toasted almonds and arugula into small pieces. Add them to the pan and cook for another minute.

Now add the boiled millet, stir gently and serve as you like. If you want to present it the way I did, you need to use an aluminium bowl or a cup, moisten the inside, fill it with the millet and mash well. Then invert onto a serving plate and decorate as desired.

Millet with arugula pesto

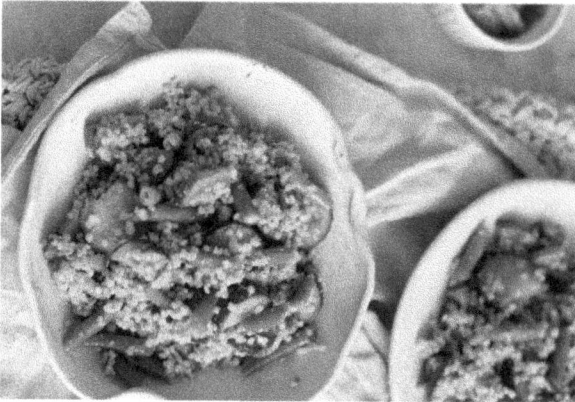

Ingredients for 2 people:

~ 1 cup hulled millet
~ 100 g of rocket
~ 60 g of almonds
~ 2 teaspoons of capers
~ 1 teaspoon of mustard
~ 1/2 loaf of natural tempeh
~ 2 spring onions
~ 2 tablespoons rice acidulate or apple cider vinegar
~ 2 tablespoons rice malt
~ 1 tablespoon tamari or shoyu (soy sauce)
~ aigrette
~ umeboshi acidulate
~ orange or lemon juice

Instructions

Wash the millet well and boil it 10-15 minutes with twice the volume of water and a pinch of salt.

At the end of the cooking time turn off the flame and let it rest covered for 10 minutes. There are various types of millet that differ in cooking time. Some take as long as 20 minutes.

Find your favorite millet and discover the perfect cooking time.

Pulverize 40 g of almonds and blend them with the arugula, capers, mustard, a little oil and if necessary a little water. Adjust the salt.

To avoid damaging the arugula with the heat of the blades and to accentuate the bitter taste, you can add an ice cube while blending.

Cut the tempeh into cubes and sauté in a pan with a little oil for 5 minutes.

Slice the spring onion and add it to the tempeh. Sauté for 1 minute and deglaze with vinegar.

Add the tamari and malt and let caramelize over medium heat.

Bake the remaining almonds at 160° for 10-15 minutes, to toast them.

Blanch the aigrette in boiling salted water for a few minutes, let them cool and season with the rice vinegar, umeboshi acidulate and lemon or orange juice.

Remove the almonds from the oven and cut them into strips to add to the aigrette.

Millet with peas and dried daikon

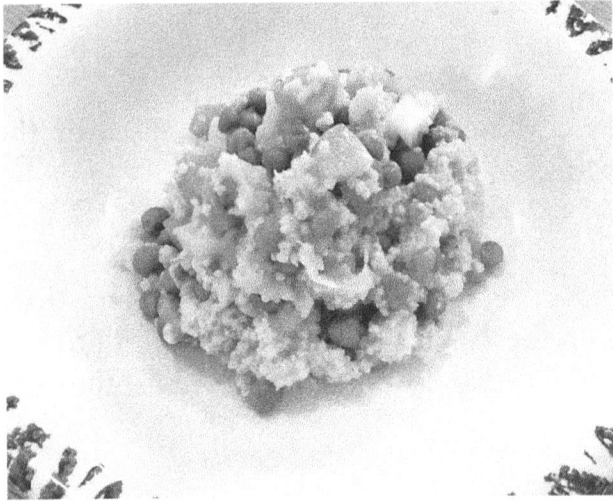

Stir the millet into the pan with the vegetables and serve with a sprinkle of gomasio.

Ingredients

- ~ 1 cup of husked millet
- ~ 1 onion
- ~ 1 handful of dried daikon
- ~ 1 cup cooked peas
- ~ 1 tablespoon oil
- ~ 2 tablespoons shoyu or tamari (soy sauce)
- ~ 1 mint leaf
- ~ gomasio

Instructions

Wash the millet well and boil it with double or triple the volume of water and a pinch of salt for 10-15 minutes. At the end of cooking, when the water is almost completely absorbed, turn off the heat and let rest covered. Soak the dried daikon for 10 minutes. In the meantime, slice the onion and stew it in a pan with oil and a little water. Add the dried daikon and cook for 10 minutes. When cooked, add the peas, shoyu or tamari and mint strips and cook for another 2 minutes.

Second Courses

Adzuki and leek patties

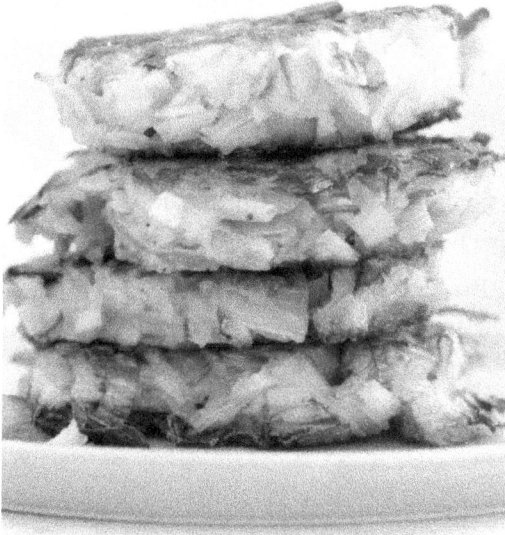

Ingredients for about ten patties:

~ 100 g cooked azuki
~ ½ leek
~ 1 sprig of rosemary
~ 1 sprig of thyme
~ 1-2 tablespoons soy yoghurt
~ 1 tablespoon of cornflour (or more)
~ extra virgin olive oil
~ whole sea salt
~ 1 tablespoon soy sauce

Instructions

Slice the leek finely and wilt it in a pan with 1 tablespoon of oil and 1 pinch of salt.

Chop the rosemary and add it to the pan with the thyme leaves. Add a little water if necessary.

While the leeks are cooking, blend the beans with a tablespoon of oil, 1 tablespoon of soy sauce, 1 tablespoon of yogurt.

Add the cooked leeks and 1 tablespoon of flaked cornmeal, mix well and rate the consistency.

If it allows you to make patties out of it with your hands that's fine, otherwise adjust the consistency by adding more yogurt if the mixture is too hard or flakes, or more cornmeal if it's too soft.

I like to leave the leeks in small pieces, but if you like an even consistency, you can blend the leeks, once cooked, along with the azuki.

Heat a skillet brushed with oil and brown the patties on both sides.

You can serve with a fresh salad.

Mini burgers of legumes

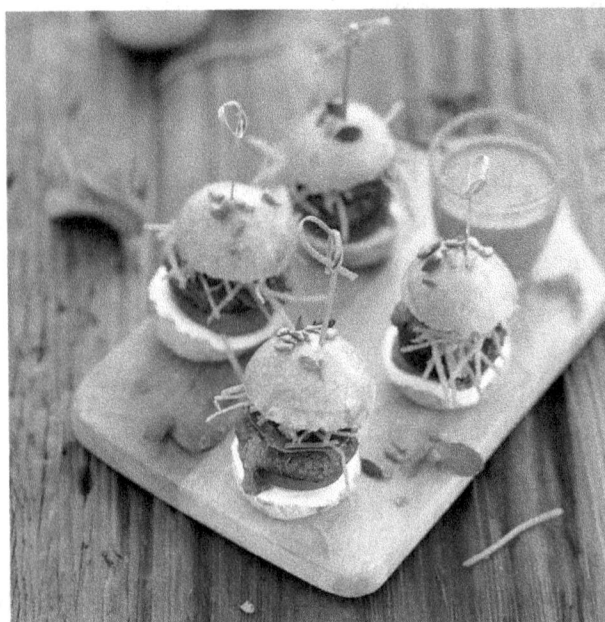

Slice the onion and carrot and cook in a pan with oil, a little water and a pinch of salt. Cook the cereal flakes with 1 cup of water for 10-15 minutes until the water has evaporated. Blend the pulses with the cooked vegetables, cereal flakes, chopped pistachios, chopped parsley, thyme, spices and salt.

Transfer the mixture to a bowl and add a handful of sunflower seeds and some breadcrumbs to make a soft, yet firm dough. Wrap the dough with plastic wrap forming a roll and refrigerate 2 hours or place in the freezer for 15 minutes. The diameter of the roll will determine the size of the burgers.

Remove the foil and slice the roll and cook the burgers in a skillet, oven or grill. Serve with a sprinkle of gomasio or various seeds, such as poppy, alpha-alpha, etc., accompanied by vegetables.

Ingredients

~ 200 g of boiled legumes
~ 80 g of oatmeal or barley flakes (better if whole grain)
~ 30 g of unsalted shelled pistachios
~ 1 onion
~ 1 carrot
~ Sunflower seeds
~ ½ teaspoon of curry
~ 1 pinch of cumin
~ 1 pinch coriander
~ oregano, thyme, parsley
~ 2 teaspoons salt
~ breadcrumbs
~ 2 tablespoons extra virgin olive oil

Instructions

You can make these burgers with any legumes you like, beans, lentils, azuki, chickpeas, etc.

Chickpea croquettes

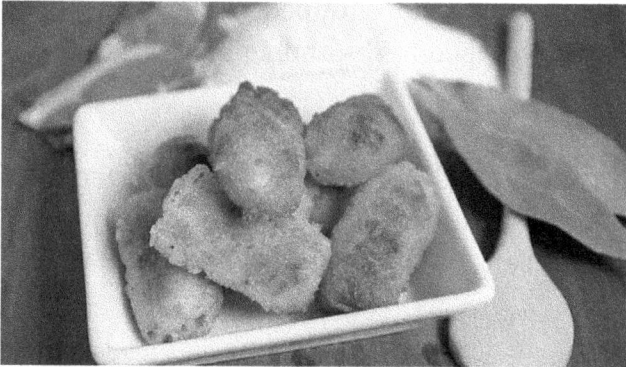

~ **Ingredients for about 40 small croquettes:**
~ 1 large onion
~ 250 g of boiled chickpeas
~ 2 tablespoons chickpea flour or brown rice flour
~ 2 tablespoons oil
~ 2 tablespoons shoyu or tamari (soy sauce)
~ rosemary
~ thyme
~ ½ teaspoon sweet curry
~ cornflour
~ whole sea salt

Instructions

Slice the onion thinly and sauté it in a pan with the oil, a pinch of salt and the curry powder. Add the boiled chickpeas, shoyu, chopped rosemary, thyme leaves and a little water to stew until the onions are cooked.

Blend the onions and chickpeas well and add the corn-starch. If necessary, add a little corn flour, just enough to obtain a sufficiently compact but soft consistency to form croquettes with your hands.

Bread the croquettes in the corn flour.

There are two ways to cook them, either in a skillet with a little oil to brown them, or by deep frying.

If you want to make them in a pan, to make them lighter, it is better to give the croquettes a flattened shape, if instead you want to fry them in immersion (recommended, very good), it is better to give the croquettes a ball or cylinder shape.

Let cool before serving accompanied by a fresh salad. I used arugula, dandelion, valerian and sprouts.

Rice croquettes with yogurt sauce

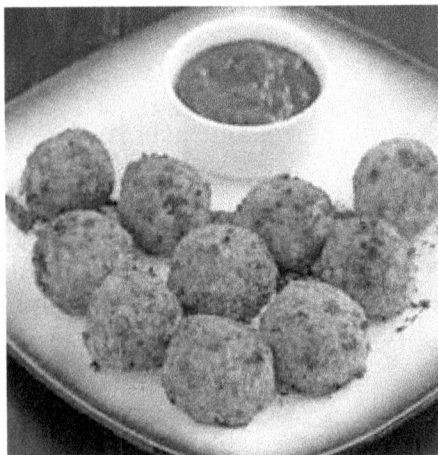

Ingredients for the croquettes

- ~ 1 glass of brown rice
- ~ 1 onion
- ~ 2 spoons of capers
- ~ 2 tablespoons of extra virgin olive oil
- ~ aromas (rosemary, thyme, savoury, sage, basil)
- ~ semi-integral flour
- ~ corn flour or breadcrumbs
- ~ evo oil

For the yogurt sauce

- ~ 150 g unsweetened soy yoghurt
- ~ 2-3 drops of umeboshi acidulate
- ~ 1 garlic clove
- ~ mint
- ~ dill
- ~ whole sea salt

Instructions

Boil the rice and sauté the onion in a pan. Add cooked rice, herbs and desalted and chopped capers. Sauté everything for a few minutes.

Cut a slice off the garlic clove and chop it finely. Prepare the sauce by blending the yogurt with the chopped garlic, umeboshi, finely chopped herbs and a pinch of salt.

Taste and add salt if necessary. Refrigerate. If you like you can add a grated and squeezed cucumber.

With wet hands, prepare some croquettes and dip them in a rather liquid batter prepared with water and flour. Dip them in corn flour and fry on both sides.

Alternatively, you can dip them only in cornmeal and then in a pan greased with oil or in the oven.

Serve the croquettes accompanied by the sauce.

Cubes of tofu with saffron

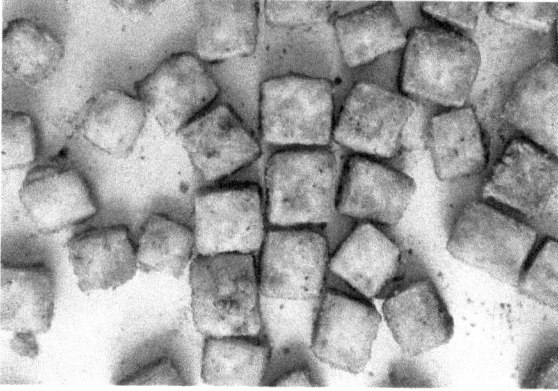

Ingredients for about 20-30 cubes of tofu:

- ~ 180-200 g of natural tofu
- ~ 1 sachet of saffron
- ~ 100 g semi-whole wheat flour type 1 or type 2
- ~ ½ teaspoon of natural yeast (cream of tartar)
- ~ parsley for garnish
- ~ tamari or shoyu
- ~ oil for frying (it would be better to use evo oil)
- ~ toothpicks

For the spicy pyramids

- ~ 150-200 g fresh daikon or radish)
- ~ a piece of fresh ginger root
- ~ 1 teaspoon of umeboshi acidulate

Instructions

Cut the tofu into cubes about 2 cm thick and transfer to a bowl. Pour in some soy sauce (5-6 tablespoons) and a little water, enough to cover the cubes and let them marinate for 2-3 hours.

Clean the daikon and grate it finely. Squeeze out the pulp and set aside. Grate the ginger to get about a teaspoon of pulp and mix it with the daikon. Add the sour cream, mix and form pyramids (or other shapes) with your hands to go with the skewers. If you like you can also add wasabi powder or paste.

After the necessary time has elapsed, prepare a batter by combining in a bowl the flour, yeast, saffron and enough water to form a thick batter.

Heat plenty of oil in a frying pan and in the meantime prepare the tofu cubes by piercing each one with a toothpick.

Dip them in the batter and dip them in the hot oil for a few minutes until they are golden brown. Let them cool on absorbent paper and serve accompanied by the spicy pyramids and a sprinkling of chopped parsley.

Tofu with four roots

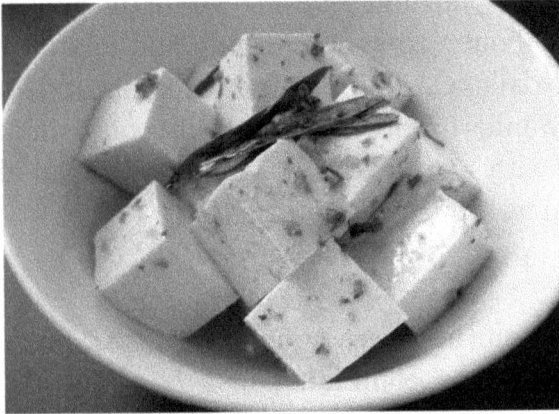

Ingredients

- ~ 100 g of natural tofu
- ~ a handful of lotus root slices
- ~ a handful of burdock sticks
- ~ 2 small onions or 1 large
- ~ 2 carrots
- ~ 2 tablespoons extra virgin olive oil
- ~ 4 tablespoons of tamari
- ~ 1 tablespoon ginger juice
- ~ 1 tablespoon umeboshi acidulate

Instructions

Dice the tofu and let it marinate for about 20 minutes in a mixture of 2 tablespoons of tamari (or shoyu), the ginger juice, umeboshi acidulate and a little water.

Soak the lotus root and burdock root in warm water.

Meanwhile, slice the onion thinly and cut the carrot into small pieces. Put the onion in a pan with oil and a little water and let it brown. When the burdock and lotus are soft, remove them from the soaking water (which you can use for cooking).

Cut the lotus root into small pieces and add it to the pan with the burdock and carrots. If you want to leave the lotus root in rounds to take advantage of the "scenic" effect, you will need to calculate longer cooking times (even half an hour).

At this point the tofu should be fairly marinated. Drain it from the marinating liquid (which you can use in part for cooking) and add it to the pan with the vegetables. Add a little water (or some of the marinade) and let stew covered for 15 minutes.

Add 2 tablespoons of tamari (or shoyu) and cook for another minute. Serve hot.

Tofu with vegetables and hiziki

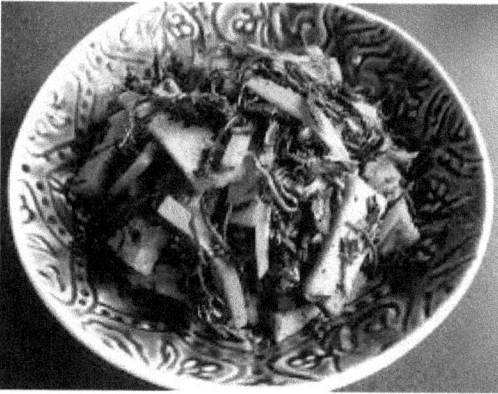

Ingredients

- ~ 1 loaf of natural tofu
- ~ 1 onion
- ~ 2 dried shitake mushrooms
- ~ 2 tablespoons of extra virgin olive oil or sesame oil
- ~ 2 tablespoons of tamari or shoyu (soy sauce)
- ~ 1 handful of hiziki seaweed
- ~ 2-3 mint leaves
- ~ 2 tablespoons apple cider vinegar
- ~ 1 teaspoon umeboshi acidulate
- ~ 1/2 teaspoon ginger juice (or more, to taste)
- ~ gomasio to taste

Instructions

Soak the seaweed and mushrooms for 15-20 minutes.

In the meantime, slice the onion and brown it in a pan with the oil, 1-2 tablespoons of water and a pinch of salt.

When the mushrooms are soft, remove the stalks, slice them and add them to the pan. Sauté 1-2 minutes, stirring, and add the diced tofu.

Add a little water and cook covered for 10-15 minutes. When cooked, add the tamari or shoyu and cook for another 1 minute.

Transfer seaweed to a pan and cover with water. Add vinegar and bring to a boil. Cook uncovered for about 20 minutes until the water is almost completely absorbed.

Season with sour cream, ginger juice, mint leaves cut into strips and gomasio.

Serve the tofu with vegetables accompanied by the hiziki.

Ginger tofu with pan-fried vegetables

You can make this dish using any seasonal vegetables you like.

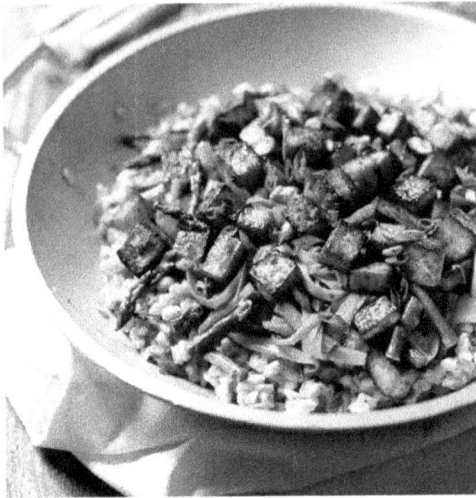

Ingredients

- ~ 1/2 loaf of natural tofu
- ~ tamari or shoyu (soy sauce)
- ~ various flavourings (rosemary, sage, etc.)
- ~ 1/2 leek
- ~ 1 carrot
- ~ a handful of radicchio
- ~ 1 tablespoon extra virgin olive oil
- ~ 1 teaspoon of ginger juice
- ~ fresh sprouts

Instructions

Cut tofu into small cubes and marinate with tamari, ginger juice and various flavourings for at least 30 minutes. Thinly slice the leek and carrots and sauté 2 minutes in oil.

Add the tofu and radicchio strips and cook for 5 minutes. Add a little tamari if necessary. Add the sprouts and the dish is ready.

Tofu triangles with onion marinade

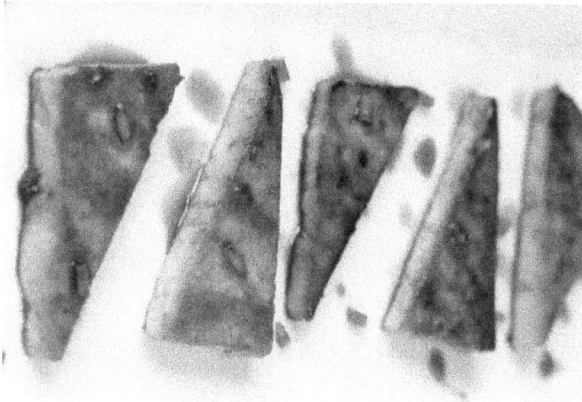

Remove the triangles from the marinade and cook them on the grill or in a pan with a little oil, browning them on both sides. Accompany the triangles with the remaining marinade.

Ingredients

- ~ 1 package of natural tofu (about 200 g)
- ~ 2 onions
- ~ 2 tablespoons of umeboshi puree
- ~ 2 tablespoons mirin (optional)
- ~ 4 tablespoons tamari or shoyu (soy sauce)
- ~ 1 tablespoon ginger juice
- ~ water
- ~ extra virgin olive oil or sesame oil

Instructions

Finely chop the onion. Prepare a mixture of ginger juice, tamari or shoyu, umeboshi puree, mirin and 4-5 tablespoons of water. Add chopped onion and slice tofu less than 1 cm thick.

Cover the tofu with the marinade and let it sit for a few hours. If it's very hot, also in the refrigerator.

Baked Tempeh

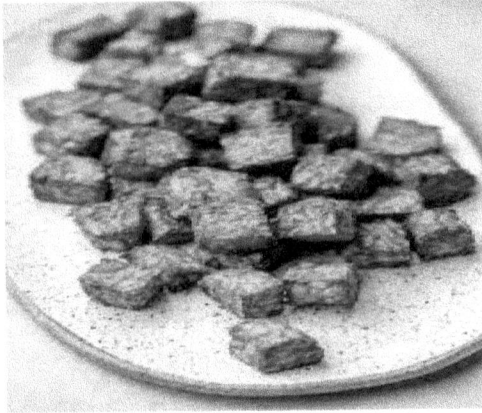

Ingredients

~ 1 loaf of natural tempeh
~ 2 tablespoons of tamari or shoyu (soy sauce)
~ 2 tablespoons of oil
~ chopped rosemary and sage

Instructions

Cut the tempeh into not too thin slices and season with oil, tamari and chopped sage and rosemary. The amount of tamari is subjective, depending on how much flavor you want to add. If you like you can add a splash of rice vinegar.

Place the tempeh on a baking sheet lined with parchment paper and bake at 180 degrees for 20 minutes. If you want it to get crispier, just leave it in the oven a little longer.

Tempeh in pan with broccoli

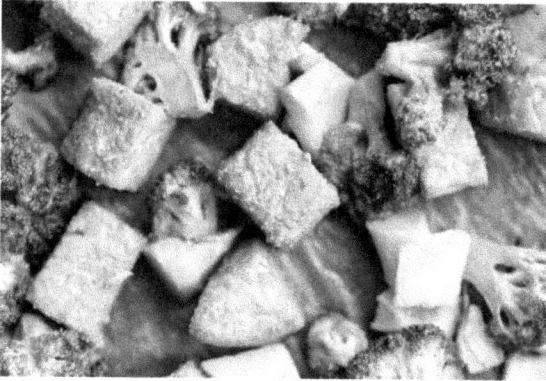

Prepare the sauce by mixing the mustard with the vinegar, umeboshi acidulate, malt and a little water.

Place the tempeh in a small bowl and add a pinch of nori seaweed flakes.

Ingredients

- ~ 1 loaf of natural tempeh
- ~ 1/2 broccoli (or a whole one, depending on your hunger!)
- ~ 1 pinch of whole sea salt
- ~ 3 tablespoons extra virgin olive oil
- ~ 1 pinch of nori seaweed flakes (optional)
- ~ 1 scant teaspoon of mustard
- ~ 1 teaspoon of umeboshi acidulate
- ~ 1 teaspoon of rice or barley malt
- ~ 1 teaspoon rice vinegar (or half of apple vinegar)
- ~ water

Instructions

Clean the broccoli, divide it into florets and steam or boil it in water.

In the meantime, cut the tempeh into cubes and sauté in a pan with the oil and salt for at least 10 minutes, until dry and golden brown.

Seitan with leeks

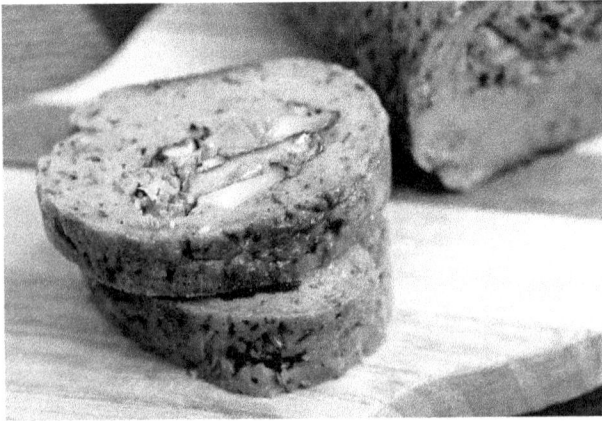

When cooked, add the ginger and sprouts and turn off the heat.

Serve garnished with a few drops of balsamic cream. This ingredient is not indispensable and can be substituted with 2 teaspoons of rice vinegar (or 1 apple vinegar) and 1 teaspoon of rice malt.

Ingredients

~ 1 leek
~ 120 g of seitan
~ 2 tablespoons of extra virgin olive oil
~ 2 tablespoons of shoyu
~ 1 teaspoon of nori seaweed flakes (optional)
~ 1 teaspoon of ginger juice
~ 2 teaspoons of balsamic vinegar cream (optional)
~ a handful of fresh sprouts
~ whole sea salt

Instructions

Slice the leek thinly wilt it in a pan with the oil and a pinch of salt. I left it a little long and it was a little fibrous, so I recommend chopping it into small pieces or rounds.

Cut the seitan into sticks or whatever shape you prefer and add it to the pan when the leek is well cooked. Add the shoyu, balsamic cream and nori seaweed and cook for a few more minutes.

Seitan escalopes with lemon

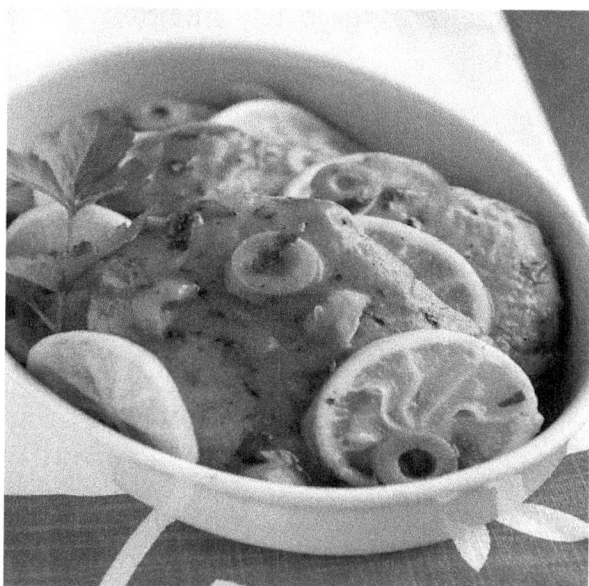

Grate the lemon peel and squeeze the juice from half the lemon.

Mix 2-3 tablespoons of lemon juice with the soy sauce, water and add the grated peel.

Cut a slice of lemon (the half not squeezed) not too thin, about half an inch.

With a knife remove the peel and cut the pulp into cubes.

Add the liquid obtained by mixing the various ingredients to the pan and let it cook for about 1 minute, until it thickens a little.

Serve with a sprinkling of chopped parsley and a few lemon cubes.

Ingredients

~ 120 g of seitan
~ 3 tablespoons extra virgin olive oil
~ 1 tablespoon of soy sauce
~ 1 lemon
~ 4-5 spoons of water
~ flour
~ parsley

Instructions

Slice the seitan thinly. There is a trick to be able to slice it thinly easily: keep the blade of the knife wet.

Flour well the "escalopes" obtained.

Heat the oil in a large, low frying pan. When it is hot, add the floured escalopes and let them brown for a few minutes, turning them on the other side.

Bites of seitan with almonds

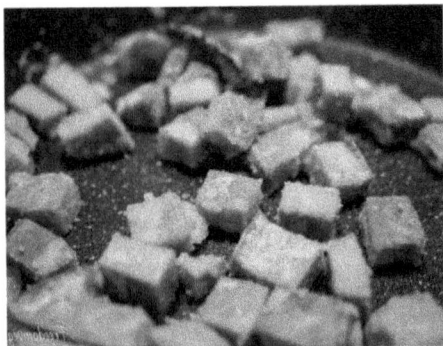

Ingredients for about 2 people:

- ~ 250 g seitan
- ~ 1 large or 2 small onions
- ~ 80 g of almonds
- ~ 1 tablespoon of ginger juice
- ~ 2 tablespoons extra virgin olive oil or sesame oil
- ~ 2-3 tablespoons of tamari or shoyu
- ~ wholemeal flour or "0" flour
- ~ 1 pinch of salt

Instructions

Spread the almonds in a baking dish lined with parchment paper and bake for about 10 minutes at 160 degrees. When you begin to smell the scent of roasted almonds will be ready. Be careful not to burn them.

Chop the onion and brown it in a pan with oil and a pinch of salt.

In the meantime, cut the seitan into cubes and flour them well.

When the onion is wilted, add the seitan and brown it for a few minutes, stirring. Add a little water and cook for a few minutes, stirring occasionally.

Do not get distracted because the presence of flour tends to make the pan stick and burn.

Add the tamari or shoyu, ginger juice and toasted almonds.

I remind you that to make ginger juice, simply grate a small piece of fresh root and then squeeze out the pulp.

If necessary, add a little more water in order to obtain a sufficient amount of juice. Stir well and it's ready.

Spoons of fennel with seitan

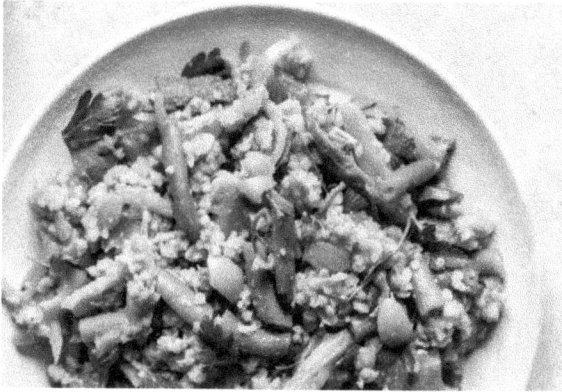

Chop the onion and dice the leftover fennel and seitan. Brown everything in a pan with the 3 tablespoons of oil. Add the raisins, pepper and a pinch of salt, mix and leave to stew covered for 5 minutes. If necessary add a little water.

At the end of the cooking time add the chopped walnuts and the whole pine nuts.

Stuff the spoonfuls of fennel with the mixture and transfer to a baking tray lined with greaseproof paper. Add a drizzle of oil, sprinkle with gomasio and cornflour (or breadcrumbs) and bake at 180° for 10-15 minutes.

Ingredients

- ~ 2 fennels
- ~ the juice of half a lemon
- ~ 1 onion
- ~ 150 of seitan or tempeh
- ~ 15 g of walnut kernels
- ~ 20 g of raisins soaked for a few minutes
- ~ 1 handful of pine nuts
- ~ 1 pinch of whole sea salt
- ~ 1 pinch of white pepper (optional)
- ~ gomasio
- ~ 3 tablespoons of extra virgin olive oil
- ~ cornflour or breadcrumbs

Instructions

Cut the bottom of the fennel and then cut it in half lengthwise so that you can get 1 or 2 "spoons" from each half. With two fennel halves I got 5 tablespoons of different sizes. Keep aside what is left over from the fennels.

Wash the "spoons" well under water and blanch them in boiling salted water acidulated with lemon juice for about 5 minutes. Remove them from the water and set them aside.

Seitan sauce

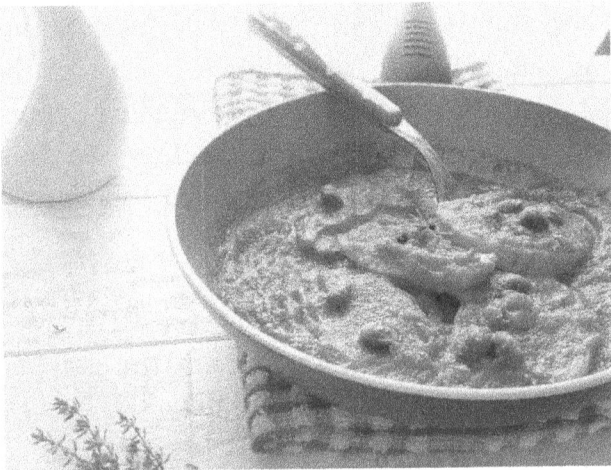

Ingredients

- ~ 200 g of seitan
- ~ 300 g of tomato puree
- ~ mixture for stir-fry (carrot, onion, celery)
- ~ garlic
- ~ rosemary
- ~ 2-3 tablespoons of oil
- ~ shoyu or tamari (soy sauce)
- ~ ½ glass of white wine (optional)

Instructions

Sauté carrot, onion, celery, garlic and rosemary in oil. Chop the seitan and add it to the pan, season with soy sauce, deglaze with wine and let it evaporate over high heat. Add the tomato and cook for 15-20 minutes. If necessary, add a little water.

Seitan, unlike meat, does not need to be cooked for a long time in this type of recipe.

Chickpea omelette with onions and spicy basmati rice

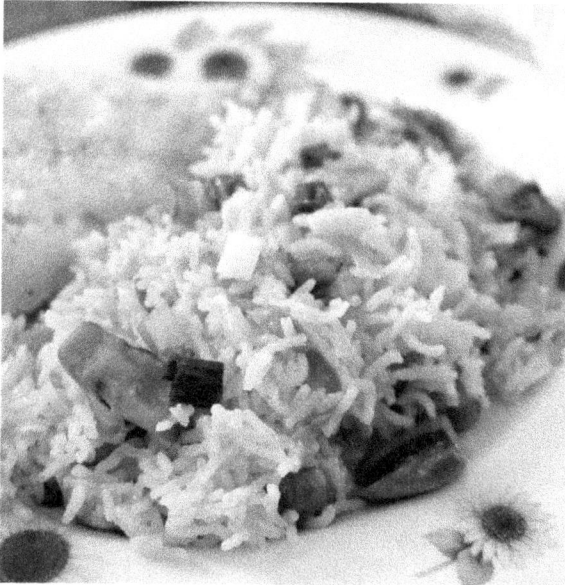

Ingredients for the omelette

- ~ 3 golden onions
- ~ 130 g of chickpea flour
- ~ 300 ml of water
- ~ 5 tablespoons of extra virgin olive oil
- ~ 2 tablespoons of tamari
- ~ whole sea salt
- ~ 1 tablespoon of oregano
- ~ Ingredients for the rice
- ~ 150 g brown basmati rice
- ~ 1 tablespoon extra virgin olive oil
- ~ 1 pinch of integral sea salt
- ~ 1 sachet of saffron
- ~ 1 teaspoon of sweet curry
- ~ 1 pinch of cumin

Instructions

Mix the chickpea flour with the water and let it sit for 30 minutes.

Thinly slice the onions and stew them in a pan with 1 tablespoon of oil, the shoyu and a little water, for about 15 minutes, or until soft.

Add ½ teaspoon of salt, the oregano and 4 tablespoons of oil to the chickpea batter. Mix well and then add the warm onions. Mix and pour into a baking dish lined with parchment paper. Make sure that the mixture is quite low, about 1 cm.

Bake for 40 minutes at 170-180°.

Meanwhile, prepare the rice. Wash it and cook it with twice the volume of water and salt. Cook semi-covered for about 15-20 minutes. At the end of cooking the water will be almost completely absorbed, turn off and leave covered for 10 minutes. Pour the rice into the pan and add the oil, the saffron dissolved separately, the curry powder and the cumin crushed or chopped with a knife.

Over medium-high heat, stir well for 5 minutes to dry the rice and toast the spices. Taste and adjust salt if necessary (with salt or shoyu). I used a pastry cup to serve and decorated with two blades of chives.

Remove the pan from the oven and let the omelette cool before cutting and serving it with the rice.

Tricolor tofu soufflé

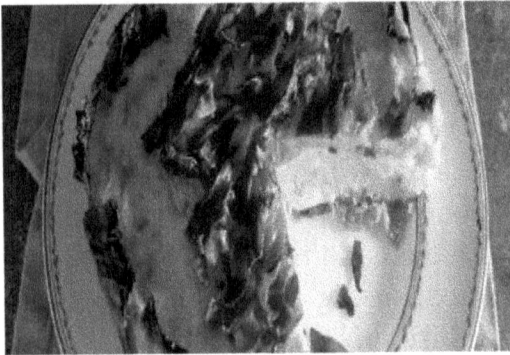

Ingredients

~ 400 g of natural tofu
~ 200 g of chard
~ 200 g of carrots
~ 200 g of cleaned pumpkin
~ 1 ½ teaspoons whole sea salt
~ ½ teaspoon cinnamon
~ ½ teaspoon nutmeg
~ 3 tablespoons extra virgin olive oil
~ 1 teaspoon agar agar powder

Instructions

Wash the chard and blanch in boiling water for 2 minutes, drain and squeeze very well. Cut the carrots and squash into small pieces and steam them.

Blend the tofu with the agar agar, salt and oil. Try to obtain a creamy consistency, so if necessary add a little water. Divide the mixture into three equal parts and blend one part with the chard, one part with carrots and nutmeg and the last part with pumpkin and cinnamon.

Line a plum-cake mold with baking paper or use the aluminium trays (greased with oil) and pour the cream of carrots, then the beets and finally the pumpkin.

Level the surface and bake at 180° for 20-30 minutes. Let cool completely, remove from the mold and decorate with poppy seeds or other decorations as desired. If you used the plum-cake mold cut into slices. Preparing it several hours in advance will keep it more compact.

Carrot flan with ginger aigrette

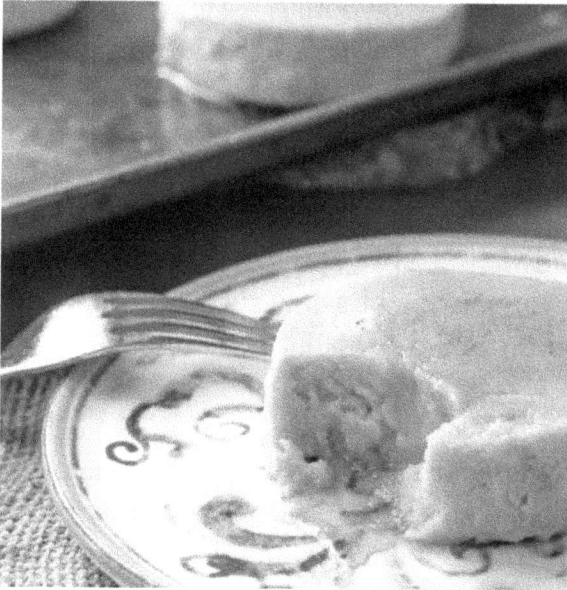

Ingredients

- ~ 5-6 carrots
- ~ 1 leek
- ~ 1 teaspoon turmeric
- ~ 1 tablespoon clear tahin
- ~ 1 teaspoon of agar agar powder
- ~ vegetable stock (carrot, celery, onion, kombu seaweed)
- ~ integral sea salt
- ~ agretti
- ~ umeboshi acidulate
- ~ ginger juice

Instructions

Prepare vegetable stock by boiling 1 onion, 1 carrot, 1 celery stalk and 2-3 cm of kombu seaweed for 15-20 min.

At the end of cooking, adjust the salt.

Cut the carrots and leek into small pieces, put them in a pot with the turmeric and agar agar and cook everything covered by the vegetable broth until almost completely absorbed.

Remove from the pot and whisk well to obtain a very smooth mixture. Combine the tahin, check for flavor and transfer to aluminium forms greased with oil.

Let cool and then unmould directly onto serving platter.

Boil the aigrette in boiling salted water and toss with the umeboshi acidulate and ginger.

Roll up some of the aigrette with a fork, like spaghetti, and place them next to the flan.

Macro-sandwich with tempeh

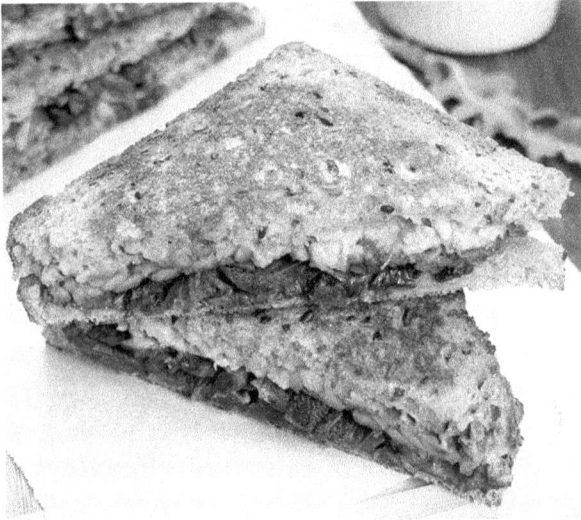

Slice the tempeh fairly thinly, dip it in tamari and then in cornmeal to bread it. Fry the breaded slices on both sides for a few minutes, until golden brown. Transfer to paper towels to cool.

Wash the salad and slice the bread. Prepare sandwich 1 by spreading a little vegan mayonnaise, add a few slices of tempeh, the sprouts and the salad.

Now prepare sandwich 2. Cut the carrot into julienne and let it soak for 10-15 minutes with a mixture of umeboshi acidulate and water (the proportion is 1:3).

In the meantime, prepare a sauce by mixing the tahin (sesame cream) with the umeboshi puree and a little water, to mix well and obtain a cream. Instead of umeboshi puree you can use lemon and salt, or miso.

Slice the olives and prepare sandwich 2 by spreading the cream, then add a few slices of tempeh, some carrots, olives and chives.

Ingredients to prepare breaded and fried tempeh:

- ~ 1/2 loaf of tempeh
- ~ corn flour
- ~ tamari or shoyu (soy sauce)
- ~ extra virgin olive oil
- ~ Bread roll 1
- ~ sourdough wholemeal bread
- ~ breaded and fried tempeh
- ~ salad to taste
- ~ vegan mayonnaise
- ~ sprouts

Sandwich 2

- ~ sourdough wholemeal bread
- ~ 1 carrot
- ~ green olives
- ~ 1 tablespoon of clear tahin
- ~ 1/2 teaspoon of umeboshi puree
- ~ chives
- ~ olives

Instructions

Side dishes, Soups and Salads

Red bean velouté

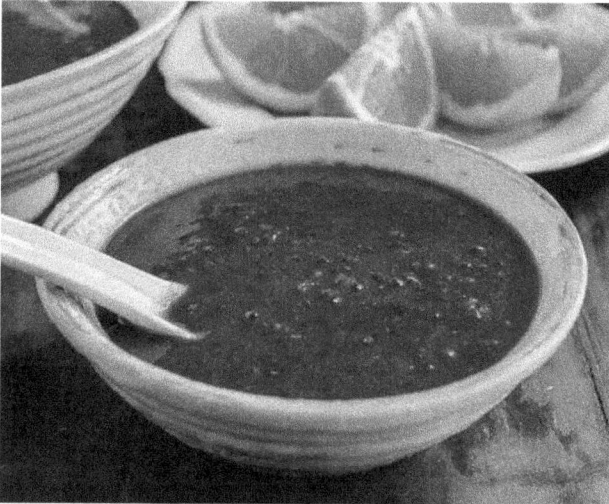

Ingredients for about 4 people:

- ~ 250 g of red beans
- ~ 1 carrot
- ~ 1 celery stalk
- ~ 1 garlic clove
- ~ half onion
- ~ 1 bay leaf
- ~ 2 of sage
- ~ 1 small sprig of rosemary
- ~ 2 tablespoons of extra virgin olive oil
- ~ whole sea salt and or soy sauce

Instructions

Soak the beans overnight or for at least 8 hours. Discard the water and put them in a pot with plenty of water. Bring to a boil and foam as soon as they make a little foam on the surface.

At this point add all the other ingredients.

Cook for about two hours.

At the end of cooking, when the beans are well cooked, pass them in the vegetable mill with a medium hole grid and pass them a second time with a small hole grid.

It is essential to do this operation when everything is still very hot.

Here is Silvana's secret: the double pass through the masher and the heat.

If the velouté is too thick you can add a little water.

You can serve it with some croutons or with a few drops of vegetable cream.

Cream of pumpkin, white turnip and curry sauce

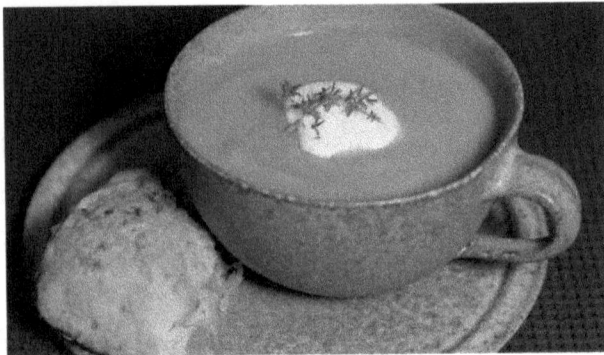

Ingredients

- ~ 1 onion
- ~ 1 white turnip (about 200 g)
- ~ 600 g pumpkin, cleaned without peel
- ~ 2 teaspoons of curry powder
- ~ 2 tablespoons extra-virgin olive oil or sesame oil
- ~ 1 teaspoon whole sea salt
- ~ 1 teaspoon of rice or barley miso
- ~ about 400 ml of water
- ~ 2 tablespoons of tamari (soy sauce)
- ~ pine nuts
- ~ chives

Instructions

Thinly slice the onion and brown it in a pan with the oil, curry, a little water and a pinch of salt.

With a small coconut brush, brush the turnip well under water so as to clean the skin well and not have to remove it.

Cut the turnip and pumpkin into small pieces and add them to the pan. Sauté for a minute then add the water, the teaspoon of salt and the tamari and bring to a boil. Cook covered for 15-20 minutes until the vegetables are soft (the time depends on the cut of the vegetables).

At the end of cooking, blend well to obtain a smooth consistency. Melt the miso separately and add it to the velouté.

Serve with chives or parsley and pine nuts to taste.

Pumpkin soup with cinnamon flavor

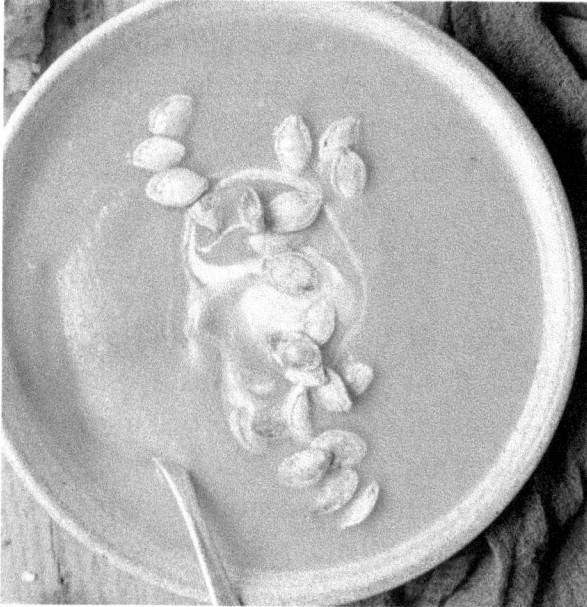

Once cooked, blend well to obtain a very smooth mixture.

Dissolve miso in 1 cup of boiling water and add it to the velouté stirring well.

Ingredients

- ~ 800 g of peeled pumpkin
- ~ 2 onions
- ~ 2 tablespoons of extra virgin olive oil
- ~ 2-3 tablespoons of shoyu or tamari (soy sauce)
- ~ 2 teaspoons of rice or barley miso
- ~ 1 pinch of cinnamon powder

Instructions

Slice the onion and brown it in a pan with the oil and a little water.

Add the chopped pumpkin and let it cook, stirring for a few minutes. Add 2 cups of water and the shoyu or tamari and let it stew, covered, for 10-15 minutes. If necessary, add more water during cooking.

Millet, lentil and turmeric soup

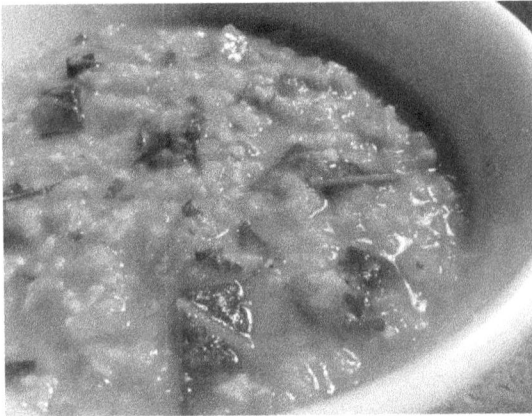

Ingredients for about 4 people:

- ~ 1 onion
- ~ 1 garlic clove
- ~ 200 g of peeled pumpkin
- ~ 1 carrot
- ~ 80 g hulled millet
- ~ 50 g hulled lentils
- ~ 1/2 teaspoon turmeric
- ~ 1 teaspoon sweet curry
- ~ 5-10 cm of wakame seaweed (or 1 tablespoon if it is in pieces)
- ~ 1 litre of vegetable stock or water
- ~ 2 sage leaves
- ~ 1 tablespoon extra virgin olive oil
- ~ 1 pinch of salt
- ~ 1 tablespoon of tamari or shoyu (soy sauce)
- ~ 1 teaspoon of rice or barley miso
- ~ 1 teaspoon of ginger juice
- ~ parsley

Instructions

Slice the onion and start browning it with the oil in the pot that will be used for the soup. Add turmeric, curry powder, salt and a little water and let it cook for a few minutes. In the meantime, clean the carrot and cut it into small pieces.

Cut the pumpkin into cubes and add it with the carrot to the pot. Also add the tamari, garlic and sage. Soak the wakame for 5 minutes. When soft, cut into small pieces and add to pot.

Add the lentils, broth or water and bring back to a boil. Cook for 10 minutes, then add the washed and drained millet. Cook another 10-15 minutes and turn off. Add the ginger juice and the miso melted separately with some of the soup. Stir well and serve with a sprinkling of chopped parsley.

Cream of brown millet with stewed leeks

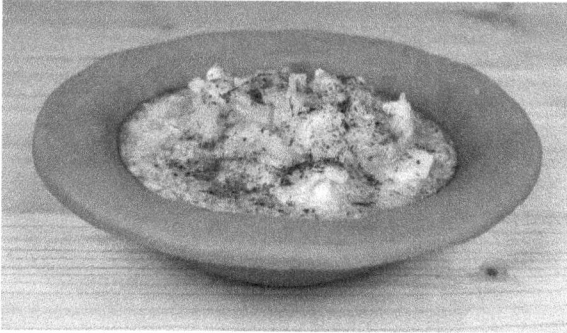

Ingredients

~ 1 litre of water
~ 1 onion
~ 1 carrot
~ 1 small daikon (optional)
~ 1 leek
~ 1 tablespoon of miso
~ 1 tablespoon tamari or shoyu (soy sauce)
~ sesame oil
~ 5 cm of wakame seaweed
~ 3 slices of dried lotus root (optional)
~ 50 g brown millet flour
~ 2 tablespoons of corn-starch or arrowroot
~ poppy seeds for decoration

Instructions

Put the water to heat and the lotus root to soak.

Peel the onion and clean the carrot and daikon with a coconut brush.

Cut these 3 vegetables into small pieces and transfer them to the pot with the water that is heating up.

As soon as the lotus root is soft, cut it into small pieces and add it to the pot.

Add the wakame seaweed (no need to soak it in this case) and cover with a lid. Let it boil for 15-20 minutes.

Meanwhile, prepare the leeks by cutting them thinly. Put them in a pan with a little oil and a pinch of salt and let them stew covered for about 10 minutes.

When cooked, add the tamari and cook for another minute.

When the broth is ready, remove the vegetables and seaweed and dissolve the millet flour and starch in a little broth. Add to the pot and cook for 1 minute, stirring.

With a little of the resulting cream, dissolve the miso on the side and add it at the end of cooking. Turn off the heat and serve the cream with some of the stewed leeks. Decorate with poppy seeds.

The vegetables used to make the broth can be recovered in other preparations or eaten directly, seasoned as desired.

An alternative to try (I didn't have time, but I encourage you to try) is to blend them well and add them to the cream of millet.

Vegetable Mayonnaise

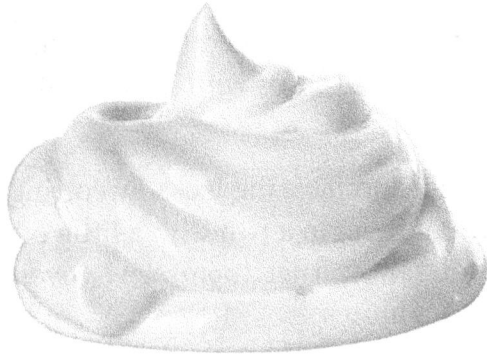

If you want to get a yellow mayonnaise, so it looks similar to the classic one, you can add 1/2 teaspoon of turmeric.

Ingredients

- ~ 100 ml of unsweetened soy milk
- ~ about 20 g of e.v.o. oil
- ~ about 40 g of sunflower or corn oil
- ~ Lemon juice to taste
- ~ ½ teaspoon whole sea salt (about 3 g)
- ~ ½ teaspoon unsweetened mustard

Instructions

In order to avoid the cooling effect of raw soy milk and to make it more digestible, it should be cooked for at least 10 minutes and then allowed to cool down. It is not essential of course, but it is recommended, especially if you suffer from reflux and colitis.

When cold, blend it with the lemon juice, mustard and salt.

Add the oils and blend again. If it doesn't whip enough add a little more oil.

Puree of broad beans with mint and lemon

Serve on croutons or to accompany cereal or croquettes.

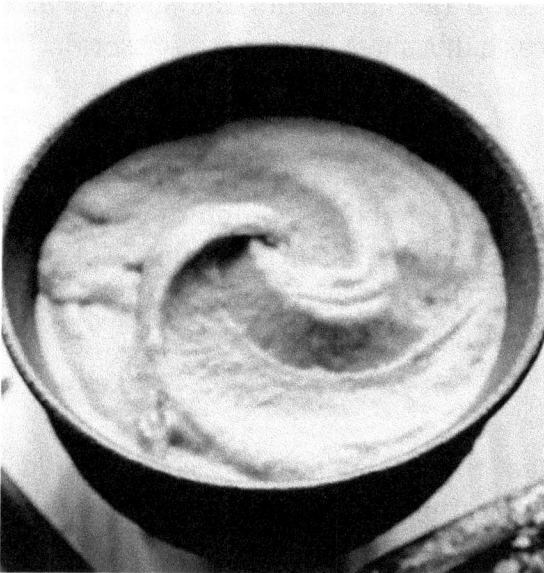

Ingredients

- ~ 200 g of shelled fresh broad beans
- ~ 1 small onion
- ~ the juice of half a lemon
- ~ 5-6 mint leaves
- ~ 2 tablespoons of extra virgin olive oil
- ~ 1 tablespoon of tamari or shoyu (soy sauce)

Instructions

Blanch the fava beans in salted water for 2 minutes. Transfer them to cold water and peel them. Put the fava beans in a pan with the finely chopped onion, oil, a little water and cook for 15-20 minutes until the fava beans are well cooked. Add the shoyu and cook another 2 minutes. Blend the fava beans with the mint and lemon juice.

Soup saves liver

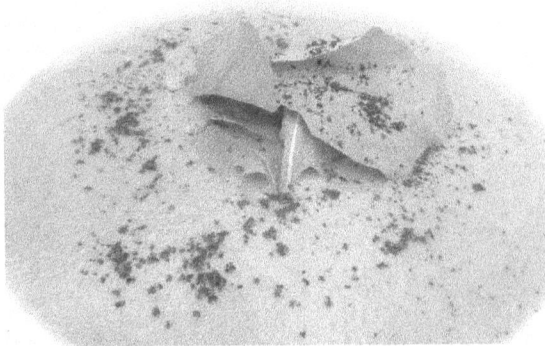

Ingredients

- ~ 1 litre and a half of water
- ~ 1 piece of leek (about 50 g)
- ~ 1 piece of daikon (about 150 g)
- ~ 3 cabbage leaves
- ~ 3-4 shitake mushrooms
- ~ 1 carrot
- ~ 5 cm of wakame seaweed
- ~ 1 teaspoon of nori seaweed flakes or ½ sheet
- ~ 1 umeboshi plum
- ~ 1 teaspoon of ginger juice
- ~ 1 teaspoon miso (or more, to taste)

Instructions

Put the water to heat on the stove. Soak the wakame seaweed and shitake mushrooms separately. Meanwhile, start preparing the vegetables. Slice the leek, carrot, daikon and cabbage.

When the wakame seaweed and mushrooms are soft, cut them into small pieces.

When the water boils, throw all the vegetables (including the mushrooms and wakame) into the pot. Also add the nori seaweed. If you do not have the flakes, but the sheets, cut into pieces half a sheet (even with scissors).

Bring to a boil and cook over medium heat, with a lid, for about 10 minutes. Cooking time will vary depending on how thin the vegetables are cut. The thinner they are, the less time they take to cook.

When the vegetables are cooked, add the umeboshi plum, removed from the stone and crushed with a fork. Dissolve miso with a little of the cooking water and add it to the soup.

Grate a piece of ginger root and squeeze the pulp between your fingers to extract the juice. Add about 1 teaspoon, or more, to taste.

Oatmeal, lentils and chestnuts soup

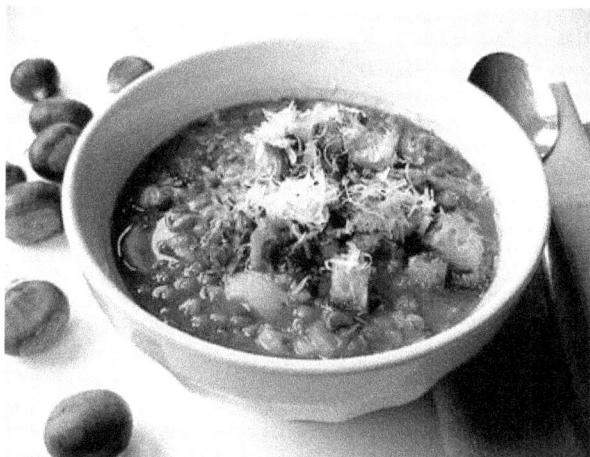

Ingredients

~ 150 of hulled oats
~ 100 g of small lentils
~ 50 g of dried chestnuts
~ 2 onions
~ 2 carrots
~ 5-6 cabbage leaves (about 100 g)
~ 2 litres of water (approx.)
~ 10 cm of wakame seaweed
~ 1 tablespoon of rice or barley miso (or more)
~ a few leaves of sage
~ 1 sprig of rosemary
~ 1 garlic clove
~ 2 tablespoons of extra virgin olive oil
~ 2 tablespoons of tamari or shoyu (or a generous pinch of salt)

Instructions

Wash the oats and let them soak for 6-8 hours along with the dried chestnuts. Wash the lentils and let them soak for 1 hour.

After the soaking time, put the oats and chestnuts in a pot with 2 litres of water and bring to a boil. Add the sage and cook for 15-20 minutes. At this point add the lentils and cook for another 15 minutes.

In the meantime, soak the wakame seaweed and start preparing the vegetables. Add the thinly sliced onions, the chopped carrots, the cabbage cut into strips and the seaweed cut into small pieces. Cook another 10 minutes.

At this point the oats, lentils and vegetables should be cooked. Add the soy sauce, oil and rosemary sprig and cook for a few more minutes.

Separately, dissolve the miso in a little of the soup liquid and add it to the soup while the heat is off. Stir well and serve hot.

If you wish, you can also add some ginger juice.

Chlorophyll broth

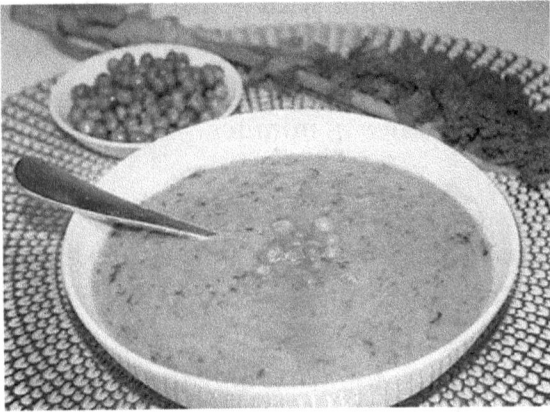

Leaves of cabbage (Savoy cabbage, cabbage, etc.), broccoli, cauliflower, leaves of carrots, radishes, leeks, turnip greens, parsley and even lettuce are all fine.

Chlorophyll broth stimulates liver function and relaxes the liver, but not only that, it promotes detoxification, helps lower cholesterol, improves cellular oxygenation, increases red blood cells and improves blood quality.

Ingredients

~ 1/2 cup chopped green leaves (I used 2 cabbage leaves)
~ 1 cup water

Instructions

Roughly chop the green leaves and boil for 1-2 minutes (without salt). Strain and drink hot.

You can drink 1-2 cups a day, best hot and on an empty stomach.

If drunk 10 minutes before meals it helps to reduce any belly bloating.

The cooked leaves can be recovered in a minestrone, vegetable stir-fry, etc.

In order to make chlorophyll broth it is necessary to use green leaves, practically all of them are good, except those of spinach and chard, too rich in calcium oxalates.

Quinoa Salad

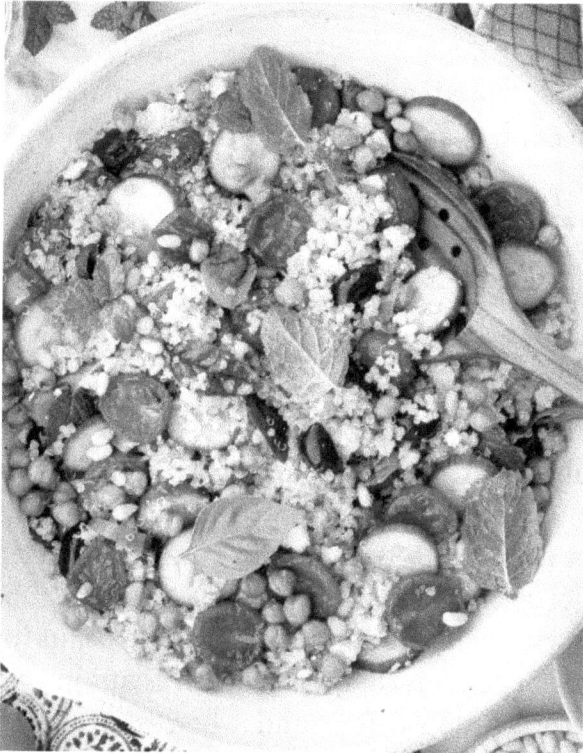

Cook for 15 minutes from the boil and at the end of cooking let rest covered for 10 minutes.

In the meantime, cut the seitan into cubes and prepare a sauce by mixing the tahini with the mustard, sour cream and vinegar. The presence of tahin, which is quite fatty, allows you to not use oil and make this salad less caloric.

When the quinoa is ready toss it with the sauce, add the seitan, capers and chopped chives.

Ingredients

- ~ 1 cup of quinoa (about 150 g)
- ~ 100 g of seitan (optional)
- ~ 1 tablespoon of tahin
- ~ ½ teaspoon of mustard
- ~ 1 tablespoon umeboshi acidulate
- ~ 1 teaspoon rice vinegar
- ~ 1 tablespoon desalted capers
- ~ 3 blades of chives
- ~ 1 pinch of whole sea salt

Instructions

Wash the quinoa and boil it with twice the volume of water and a pinch of salt.

Twice the volume means that after washing it, add 2 cups of water for cooking.

Brown rice salad

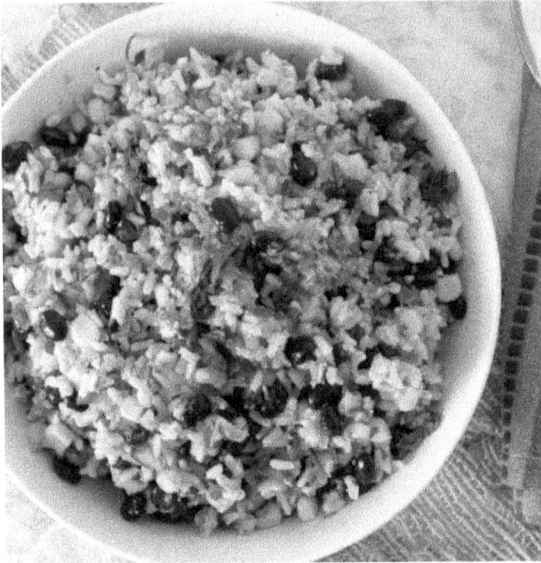

Ingredients

- ~ 150 g long-grain brown rice
- ~ 1/2 a bundle of tempeh
- ~ 4 round zucchini
- ~ 1 carrot
- ~ 1/2 daikon or 5-6 radishes
- ~ 100 g of green beans
- ~ 150 g of corn
- ~ 2 tablespoons capers
- ~ 1 tablespoon umeboshi acidulate
- ~ 2 tablespoons sunflower seeds
- ~ 2 tablespoons tamari or shoyu (soy sauce)
- ~ basil
- ~ extra virgin olive oil
- ~ poppy seeds

Instructions

Wash the rice well and let it soak overnight. Boil it with twice the volume of water and a pinch of salt for about 20 minutes with the lid on, leaving only a small gap. When the water is almost completely absorbed, turn it off and let it rest covered.

Bring salted water to a boil to blanch the zucchini 5 minutes. Cool them under water and cut off the top with the stem, without throwing it away. Now hollow out the inside with a knife and a teaspoon. Keep aside the pulp extracted, do not throw anything away!

While the rice is cooking, cut the tempeh into cubes and fry it in a pan with hot oil for 5 minutes, turning it often. When golden brown, set aside. In the same pan you can sauté the vegetables. Cut carrots and daikon into cubes (or radishes into rounds) and green beans into small cylinders. Sauté the green beans in a pan with a little oil first and when they are half cooked add the carrots and daikon. At the end of the cooking time add the diced zucchini flesh, season with tamari or shoyu or salt and cook for another minute.

When the rice is ready, let it cool or run it quickly under cold water. Add the rice to the vegetables, then add the capers, corn, basil, umeboshi and sunflower seeds. If you like you can also add a little lemon juice or ginger.

Creamy barley salad

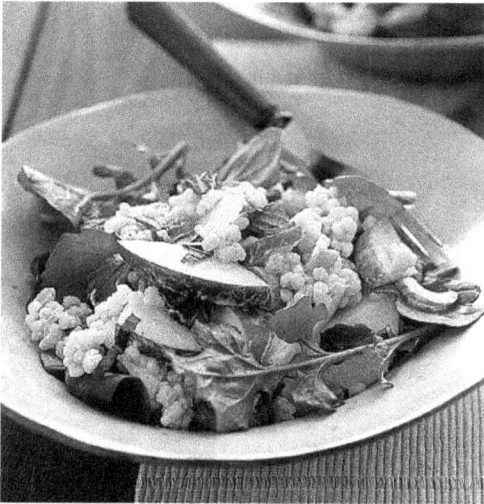

While the barley is cooking, prepare light salads of daikon and radishes, or just radishes if you can't find daikon, slicing them finely and mixing them with 1 tablespoon of umeboshi acidulate and 2-3 tablespoons of water.

Boil the tofu in water for 10 minutes. In the meantime, clean the green beans, cut them into small cylinders and sauté them in a pan with a little oil and a little water. If you like you can also add a clove of garlic that you will then remove. Cook them and season with sea salt or tamari or shoyu.

Ingredients

~ 150 g of world barley (wholemeal) or hulled barley (semi wholemeal)
~ 4-5 finely sliced radishes
~ 1/2 fresh daikon
~ 100 g of corn
~ 200 g green beans
~ 150 g natural tofu
~ 2 tablespoons umeboshi acidulate
~ 2 tablespoons of extra virgin olive oil
~ 1 tablespoon of ginger juice
~ various herbs (basil, mint, thyme)
~ tamari or shoyu (soy sauce)

Drain the tofu and plunge it into cold water to cool. Blend the tofu with 1 tablespoon umeboshi acidulate, the oil, herbs and ginger (ginger juice is extracted by squeezing the grated pulp of the fresh root). If needed, add a little water to get the consistency of a cream.

Mix the barley with the tofu cream and add the radish and daikon salads, corn and green beans. Serve warm or at room temperature.

Instructions

Wash the barley and let it soak for at least 8 hours. Boil it with 4 times the volume of water for 1 hour. At the end of cooking the water will have been completely absorbed. Turn off the heat and let it rest, covered, for 10 minutes. Pour the barley into an ovenproof dish and let it cool a little.

Artichokes stuffed with quinoa

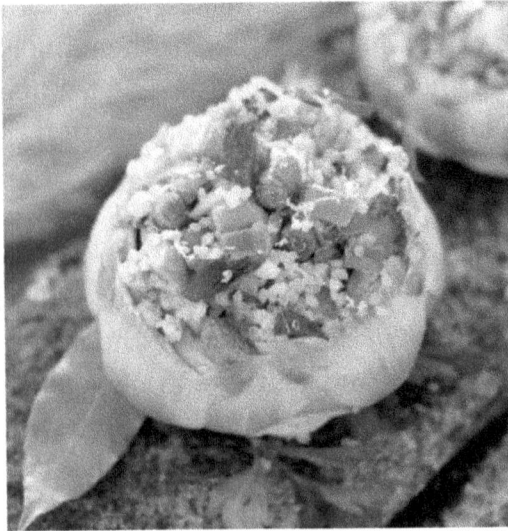

Ingredients

- ~ ½ onion
- ~ 100 g of carrots
- ~ 40 g of raisins
- ~ 4 artichokes
- ~ 70 g two-coloured or white quinoa
- ~ corn flour (optional)
- ~ 3 tablespoons extra virgin olive oil
- ~ 2-3 tablespoons of tamari or shoyu (soy sauce)
- ~ 1 pinch of whole sea salt

Instructions

Clean the artichokes. Cut them off at the base of the stem and remove the tougher outer leaves, then cut off the tip as well to make artichoke halves. Hollow out the artichokes inside with a small curved knife, to remove all the stubble and create enough cavity for you to stuff the artichokes. Place the hollowed out artichokes in a bowl with water and lemon so they don't blacken.

To shorten the cooking time in the oven, I blanched the artichokes in boiling, salted water for 3 minutes.

Clean the stems with a potato peeler and cut them into cubes. Add them to the pan with the other vegetables, to cook a few minutes.

When the quinoa is cooked and the water absorbed (even if not completely), turn off and let rest covered for 10 minutes.

Mix the quinoa with the vegetables and fill the artichokes. Move them to a baking sheet with parchment paper, sprinkle with cornmeal or breadcrumbs and drizzle with oil (about 2 tablespoons).

Bake at 190° for 20-30 minutes. Serve warm or lukewarm.

Baked cauliflower with vegan béchamel sauce

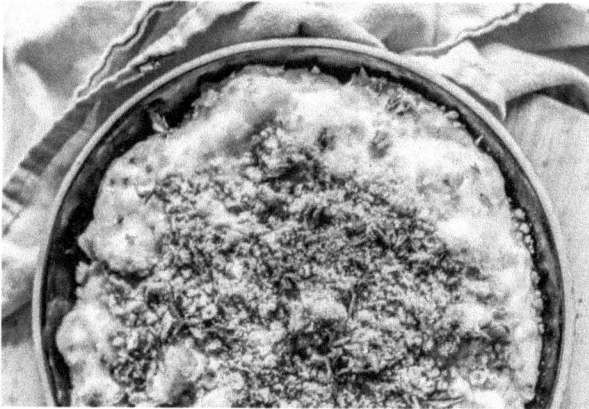

well, until you have a soft, almost liquid batter (it should slide well off the spoon).

Bring the milk to a boil and when it boils, pour in the batter, stirring with a whisk. Cook 1-2 minutes. Arrange the cauliflower on a baking sheet covered with parchment paper and pour the béchamel on top.

Sprinkle with gomasio and poppy seeds and bake for 10-15 minutes at 180°.

Ingredients

- ~ 1 cauliflower
- ~ 500 ml unsweetened soy or oat milk
- ~ 50 g of semi-whole wheat flour type 1 or type 2 (or rice flour for gluten intolerant people)
- ~ about 50 g of evo
- ~ 1 teaspoon of whole sea salt
- ~ nutmeg to taste
- ~ gomasio
- ~ poppy seeds

Instructions

Clean the cauliflower and separate the florets. I prefer to steam it leaving it al dente. If you prefer you can blanch it in boiling salted water.

Put the soy milk in a saucepan and begin to heat it over moderate heat.

In the meantime, mix the flour with the salt and nutmeg, then slowly add the oil, stirring

Pumpkin Tempura

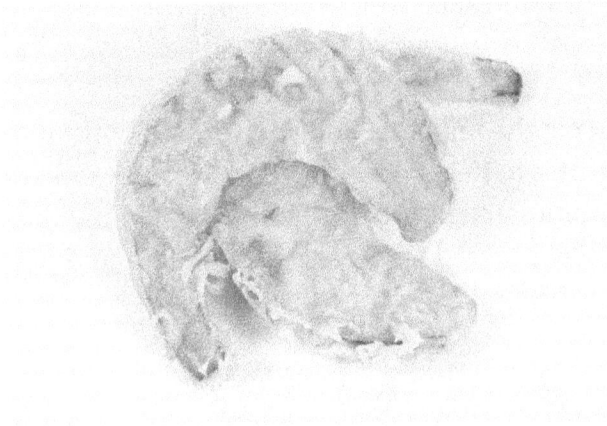

Dip the pumpkin in the batter and drop the slices into the boiling oil, frying for 2-3 minutes.

Drain well and let dry on paper towels. Tempura should be "devoured" immediately while it is hot and crispy.

Ingredients

- ~ 150 g of semi wholemeal flour type 1 or type 2
- ~ 2 tablespoons of rice starch
- ~ 1/2 teaspoon of natural yeast for cakes
- ~ 200 ml of cold water (better if carbonated)
- ~ 200 g (approx.) of cleaned pumpkin
- ~ Sesame oil
- ~ For the sauce
- ~ shoyu or tamari
- ~ lemon or ginger juice
- ~ mustard

Instructions

Prepare the sauce in which to dip the tempura, mixing shoyu or tamari with the lemon or ginger juice, a little mustard and if needed a little water. Doses are completely subjective.

Cut the squash into fairly thin slices (about 3 mm). Prepare the batter by mixing the flour, the starch and the cold water, enough to obtain a soft batter.

Adzuki and pumpkin flans

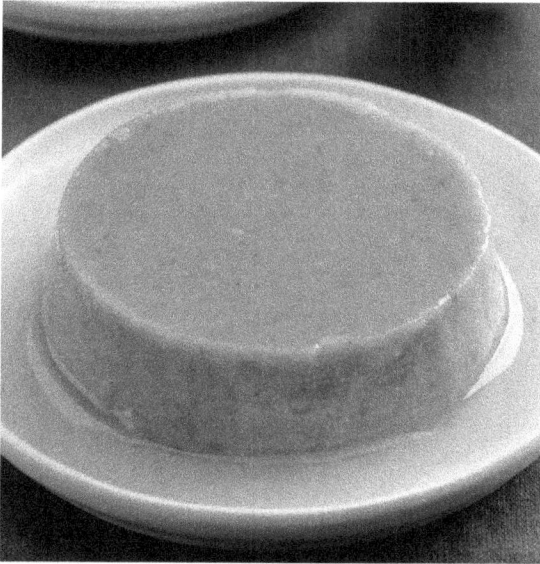

Ingredients

~ 1 onion
~ 350 g of cleaned pumpkin
~ 1 teaspoon of rice acidulate
~ 1 teaspoon umeboshi acidulate
~ 250 g of boiled adzuki beans with kombu seaweed
~ ½ teaspoon of turmeric
~ Peel of half a lemon
~ 1 sprig of thyme
~ cress seeds
~ 1 teaspoon of agar agar
~ 1 tablespoon extra virgin olive oil
~ 2 tablespoons of tamari or shoyu
~ 1 tablespoon rice miso

Instructions

Slice the onion and brown it in a pan with oil and a little water. In the meantime, cut the squash into cubes. Add the turmeric and thyme to the onions, mix well and add the pumpkin. Allow to brown for a few minutes, then add the rice vinegar and half a glass of water.

Let it stew covered for 15-20 minutes until the pumpkin is soft. If necessary, add a little more water while cooking. Add shoyu or tamari, umeboshi acidulate and agar agar dissolved separately with a little cold water. Add the azuki, dissolve the miso in a little water and add it to the pan, stirring well.

Finally, add the grated lemon peel.

Pass everything in the blender. For this preparation it is not essential to obtain a perfectly smooth mixture.

Prepare some molds or a large mold and put some watercress seeds on the bottom. Pour the mixture and bake at 180 degrees for 20 minutes. Remove from the oven and let cool perfectly before flipping. Once the mixture has solidified you can also reheat it before serving.

Savoy cabbage rolls with buckwheat

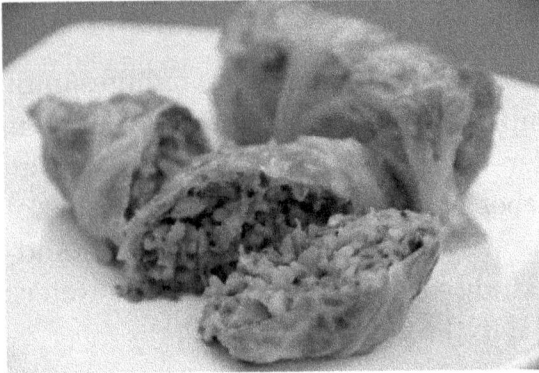

Ingredients

~ 2 carrots
~ 2 spring onions (or one onion)
~ 150 g cleaned pumpkin
~ 150 g buckwheat
~ about 10 cabbage leaves
~ 2 tablespoons extra virgin olive oil
~ whole sea salt
~ 2 tablespoons tamari
~ Vegan béchamel sauce

Instructions

Wash the buckwheat well and place it in a pot with twice the volume of water. Add a pinch of salt and bring to a boil. When it boils, lower the heat and cook partially covered for 10 minutes. When cooked, turn off the heat and leave to rest, covered, for another 10 minutes.

Divide the spring onions to separate the green part from the white part. Slice the white part and brown it in a pan with oil, salt and a little water.

Cut the carrot and pumpkin into cubes and add them to the pan. Add the soy sauce and, if necessary, a little water and let it stew for 10 minutes.

Thinly slice the green part of the spring onion and add it to the pan during the last 5 minutes of cooking.

In the meantime, blanch the savoy cabbage leaves in boiling salted water.

Add the buckwheat to the vegetables.

With the large cabbage leaves you can make two rolls, cutting them in half. With the small ones just one. Put a spoonful of buckwheat with the vegetables on half a cabbage leaf and roll it up. Then with your hands gently squeeze the roulade by tucking in the edges. You will see that it compacts. When it's ready set it aside. With 10 cabbage leaves I made 20 rolls.

Chickpea and borage pie

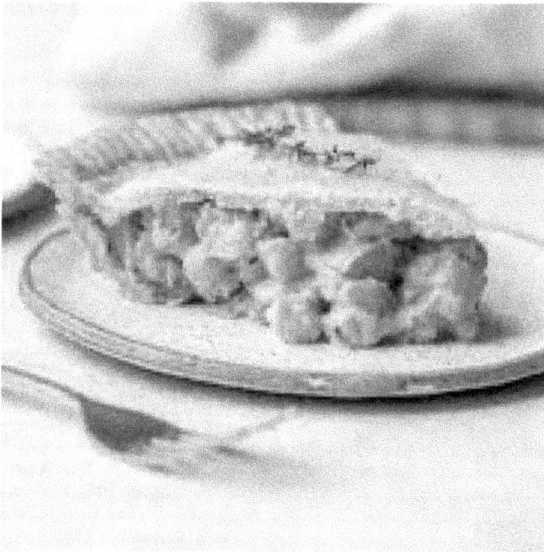

In the meantime, slice the onion thinly and brown it in a pan with 1-2 tablespoons of oil, a dash of water and a pinch of salt.

Dice the zucchini and add it to the pan with shoyu or tamari. Let it cook for a few minutes. In the meantime, wash the borage leaves well (I recommend using dishwashing gloves because some leaves sting quite a bit), cut them into strips and then into small pieces and add them to the pan. Add thyme leaves and chopped basil, stir and cook for 5 minutes.

In the meantime, mix 1/2 teaspoon of salt and 4 tablespoons of oil to the chickpea batter and prepare the mold or molds of your choice. You can use aluminium molds, greasing them with a little oil, or a small baking pan covered with parchment paper, or, as I did, a silicone mold (in this case it is not necessary to grease it).

At the end of cooking add some flowers (leave some aside for decoration) pour the vegetables into the chickpea batter, mix well and transfer to the mold.

Bake at 170-180° for about 30 minutes. Let cool well before removing from the mold and serve decorating with some flowers.

Ingredients for about 6 single-portion cupcakes:

- ~ 100 g of chickpea flour
- ~ 200 ml water
- ~ 1/2 onion or 1 shallot
- ~ 1 small zucchini
- ~ about 50 g of borage leaves (about 20 leaves)
- ~ about ten borage flowers
- ~ extra virgin olive oil
- ~ about 2 tablespoons of tamari
- ~ whole sea salt
- ~ 1 sprig of thyme
- ~ a few basil leaves

Instructions

Mix the chickpea flour with the water and let it rest for about an hour.

Adzuki with onions and rosemary

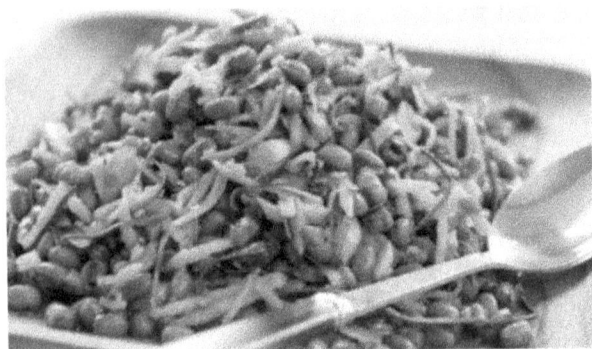

Ingredients

- ~ 100 g of dried adzuki
- ~ 2 onions
- ~ 1 sprig of rosemary
- ~ 1 tablespoon of extra virgin olive oil
- ~ 2 tablespoons of tamari or shoyu (soy sauce)
- ~ 1 piece of kombu seaweed (about 3-5 cm)

Instructions

Soak the azuki beans for 6-8 hours, change the water and cook them with the kombu seaweed for about 40 minutes. Check the cooking: they should be very soft.

Slice the onion and stew it slowly in a pan with oil and a little water.

When cooked, add the tamari and chopped rosemary. Cook for another 1-2 minutes and add the boiled beans. Stir well and serve hot or warm.

Amaranth with broad beans and ginger vegetables

Ingredients

~ 1 cup of amaranth (for about two people)
~ 2 carrots
~ 1 onion
~ 100 g of fresh broad beans removed from the pods
~ 1 teaspoon of ginger juice
~ 1 tablespoon extra virgin olive oil or sesame oil
~ 2 tablespoons tamari

Instructions

Boil the amaranth with 2 1/2 cups of water and a pinch of whole grain sea salt for about 15 minutes from boiling, covered, leaving only a small gap for steam to pass through. At the end of cooking turn off the heat and let rest covered for 10 minutes.

In the meantime scald the broad beans in boiling water for 1-2 minutes, drain and cool under water. Use a knife to cut into the skin and slide out the inside of the beans. By removing this skin they become more digestible and are suitable for even the most delicate intestines.

Slice the onion and let it brown in a pan with oil and a drop of water.

Meanwhile slice the carrots. Add the carrots and broad beans to the onions, add a little water and leave to stew covered for 10 minutes.

When cooked, add the tamari or shoyu and cook uncovered for 1 minute. Turn off the heat and add the fresh ginger juice.

You can serve the amaranth alongside the vegetables so that everyone on their own plate mixes the 2 ingredients, or you can pour the amaranth into the pan with the vegetables, mix well and serve. You can also serve it warm or at room temperature.

Desserts

Pumpkin Pudding

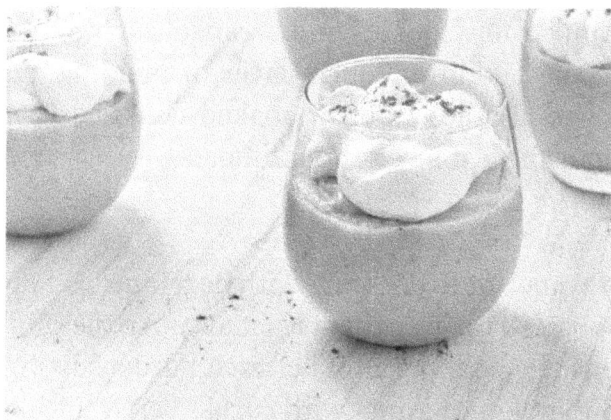

Pour the pudding into an ovenproof dish or into individual molds and allow to cool. When it is at room temperature transfer it to the refrigerator for an hour.

Cut the pudding into the shapes you prefer or remove it from the mould. Garnish to taste with almonds and rice malt or maple syrup.

Ingredients

- ~ 500 g of cleaned pumpkin
- ~ 250 ml unsweetened soy milk
- ~ 5-6 tablespoons of rice malt
- ~ 1 tablespoon of corn-starch or arrowroot
- ~ 1 level teaspoon of agar agar powder
- ~ 2 pinch of vanilla powder
- ~ 1 pinch of whole sea salt
- ~ white almonds
- ~ maple syrup (optional)

Instructions

Steam the pumpkin and when it is well cooked, transfer it to a blender. Add the milk, corn-starch, agar agar, salt and vanilla and blend well. Transfer to a small saucepan, add the malt and bring to a boil while stirring. Cook for 1 minute, stirring constantly.

Hazelnut pudding

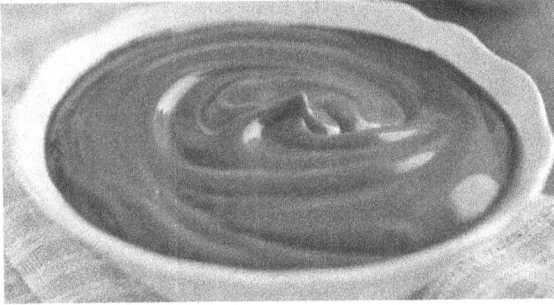

Ingredients

- ~ 500 ml of unsweetened oat milk
- ~ 1 level tablespoon of agar agar powder
- ~ 1 heaped tablespoon of corn-starch or arrowroot
- ~ 1 tablespoon of bitter cocoa
- ~ 2 generous tablespoons of hazelnut cream
- ~ 5-6 tablespoons of rice malt
- ~ 1 pinch of integral sea salt
- ~ cereal coffee
- ~ vegan dry cookies without sugar
- ~ hazelnuts for decoration

Instructions

Make the cereal coffee. I use mocha yannoh because I find it very similar to "real" coffee, so perfect for desserts. For me, a small 2 pot coffee pot was enough with the addition of a few tablespoons of water.

Dissolve the agar agar, hazelnut cream, cocoa and corn-starch in a little milk and add the rest. Add the pinch of salt and the malt and bring to a boil while stirring. The malt will dissolve well as soon as the milk heats up. As soon as the pudding is ready, let it cool no more than 1-2 minutes, stirring occasionally.

Spread some of the hazelnut pudding obtained, on the bottom of the mold or baking dish you want to use (I used a 22×16 dish).

Dunk a few cookies and arrange them on top of the pudding. Pour a layer of pudding and make another layer of soaked cookies. Then pour the last layer of pudding.

If you want to decorate with hazelnuts as I did you need to place them right away, so they sink into the pudding a bit before it hardens. If you prefer you can dust with cocoa. Serve cut into slices.

Coffee pudding yannoh

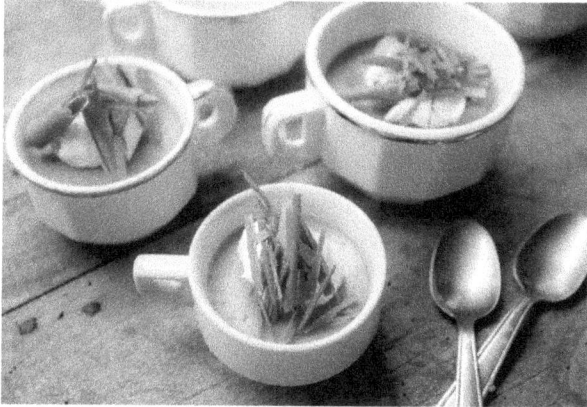

Pour the pudding into moulds or small bowls and leave to cool. When ready to serve, sprinkle with cinnamon and, if desired, dark chocolate chips.

Ingredients

- ~ 500 ml unsweetened almond milk
- ~ 1 tablespoon of soluble yannoh coffee
- ~ 2 tablespoons of brown rice flour
- ~ 4 tablespoons of rice malt
- ~ 1 pinch of whole sea salt
- ~ cinnamon powder

Instructions

Bring the milk to a boil with the yannoh coffee and a pinch of salt. Stir often and from the time of boil cook stirring for 1-2 minutes.

Strain through a fine mesh strainer and let cool. If you have soluble yannoh coffee or mocha coffee, it is not necessary to boil and filter.

Once lukewarm, mix the rice flour with a little of the coffee milk obtained, add the rest, the malt and bring back on the fire, stirring. Cook for 1-2 minutes from the boil.

Carob Pudding

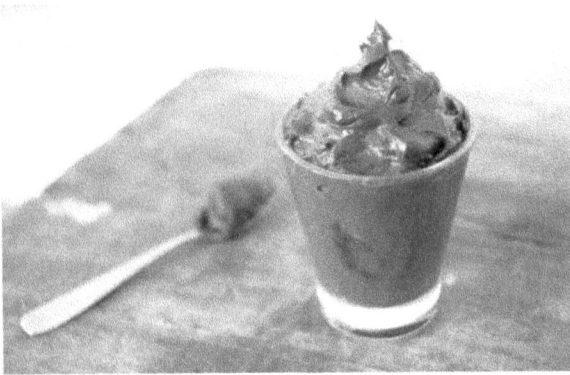

Ingredients

- ~ 500 ml of unsweetened oat milk or soy milk
- ~ 2 level tablespoons of locust bean flour (not to be confused with locust bean seed flour)
- ~ half a teaspoon of vanilla powder
- ~ 3 tablespoons brown rice flour (or rice starch)
- ~ 3 tablespoons rice malt
- ~ 1 pinch of whole sea salt

Instructions

Put the locust bean flour, vanilla, starch and salt in a small saucepan and slowly dilute with the soy milk. Add the malt, put on the heat and bring to a boil while stirring. Cook 2 minutes, stirring constantly, and pour into take-out containers or an ovenproof dish.

Decorate with pine nuts, walnuts, hazelnuts, etc., as desired.

Grape harvest pudding

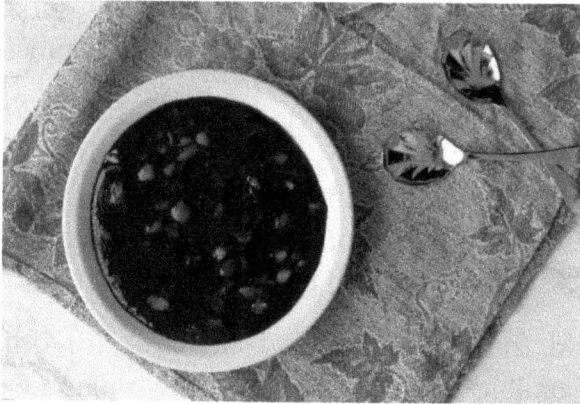

Ingredients

- ~ 500 g of black table grapes (very sweet)
- ~ 3 tablespoons rice starch
- ~ 4 tablespoons rice malt
- ~ 1 tip of teaspoon of cinnamon

Instructions

Cook grapes with 2 cups of water for 15 minutes, covered.

Puree to obtain the juice.

Dissolve the starch and cinnamon with some of the juice, stirring well with a whisk to avoid forming lumps. Add the rest of the juice and malt, mix well and bring to a simmer while stirring. Cook 1-2 minutes. Pour into cups and let cool.

Cereal Coffee Pudding

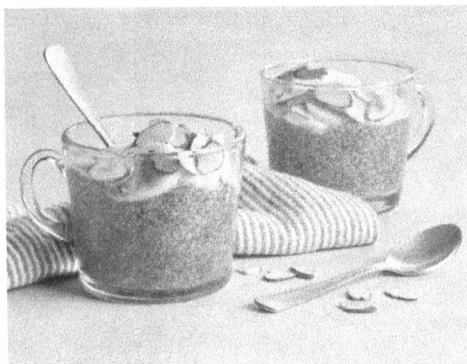

Ingredients for about 2-3 people:

For the bottom:

~ 150 g vegan cookies without butter, milk and sugar
~ 30 g of chopped hazelnuts
~ 2 tablespoons apple juice
~ 2 tablespoons rice malt

For the pudding:

~ 200 ml unsweetened soy milk
~ 120 ml unsweetened soy cream
~ 1 teaspoon of agar agar powder
~ 70-80 g of rice malt
~ ½ teaspoon of vanilla or cinnamon
~ 3 teaspoons of yannoh coffee or soluble cereals
~ 1 pinch of whole grain sea salt

For the topping:

~ 3 tablespoons rice malt
~ 2 tablespoons almond cream
~ 1 tablespoon unsweetened vegetable milk or water
~ chopped hazelnuts for garnish

Instructions

Reduce the cookies to flour and chop the hazelnuts with a knife, leaving small pieces remaining. Combine the cookies in flour with the hazelnuts, apple juice and malt. Mix well and arrange a layer in the bottom of an ovenproof dish, pressing down well. Transfer to the refrigerator and begin preparing the pudding.

In a small saucepan combine the agar agar, vanilla (or cinnamon), salt and cereal coffee (I used instant yannoh powder).

Add the soy cream and soy milk (or other vegetable milk) a little at a time, mixing well with a whisk.

Add the malt and bring to a simmer, stirring. Cook 1 minute and pour the pudding into the mold over the biscuit base.

Remember that it will only begin to set as it cools, so it is normal to remain liquid. When cooled, transfer to the refrigerator.

Prepare the topping by mixing the almond cream with the vegetable milk and malt.

When the pudding is compact and well chilled, distribute the topping and leave in the refrigerator for another half hour. You can garnish to taste with hazelnuts or dark chocolate chips. When it is well chilled, serve it cut into slices or squares.

To get the preformed single-portion, as you see in the picture, you have to use the pastry cups. Put the pastry cup on a plate or an oven dish, with a sheet of baking paper. Insert the biscuit bottoms, crushing well, and refrigerate. Pour in the pudding and let cool before transferring back to the fridge.

Add the topping and allow to cool. When ready to serve, transfer to serving platter with the help of parchment paper. Pull out from under the paper gently, lift out the ramekin and garnish as desired.

Ginger and lemon chocolates

Ingredients for about 10 chocolates

- ~ 200 g dark chocolate (I use the one sweetened with malt)
- ~ 5 cm of fresh ginger root
- ~ 2 lemons

Instructions

Grate the peel of the two lemons and set aside. Peel the ginger root and grate it, then squeeze the pulp obtained, measure out 2 teaspoons of juice and set aside.

Chop up the chocolate (with a knife or in the mixer) and melt it in a bain-marie, stirring. It is essential to melt the chocolate at a low temperature, very slowly. Patience is needed. Those who are in a hurry will end up with an unusable lump of chocolate.

When chocolate is almost completely melted add lemon peel and ginger juice. Mix well and pour the chocolate into a chocolate mold. I find silicone molds very convenient. Let cool, put in the fridge 1-2 hours and the chocolates are ready!

Ingredients

~ 300 g of pitted ripe apricots
~ 200 ml of clear apple juice
~ 2 level teaspoons of agar agar powder (about 4 g)
~ 3 tablespoons of rice malt
~ 1/2 teaspoon cinnamon (optional)
~ 1 pinch of whole sea salt

Instructions

Cut the apricots into small pieces and transfer them to a small saucepan with the apple juice, cinnamon and salt. Cook for about 10-15 minutes partially covered.

When cooked, blend well and add the malt. Dissolve the agar agar with a cup of cold water and add it to the pot stirring well with a whisk. Bring back to the heat and cook for 1 minute from the boil stirring continuously.

Pour the mixture into a mold or baking dish and let it cool. I used the silicone molds for chocolates. When cold transfer to the refrigerator for a few hours, then gently remove the jelly beans. To make them more delicious you can cover them with dark chocolate. If you use a baking dish you can cut the shape of the jellies you prefer, for example using the molds to make cookies.

They can be kept in the refrigerator for a couple of days.

Apricot and dates sorbet

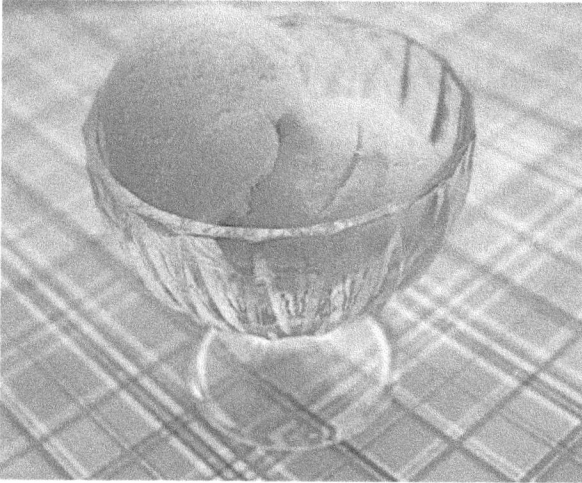

Ingredients for 5-6 sorbets

~ 4-5 fresh apricots
~ 4 dates
~ 1 tablespoon of rice malt
~ 1 teaspoon of almond cream

Instructions

Remove the apricots and dates from the stone and blend everything with the malt and almond cream.

Transfer to popsicle molds or small glasses and place in the freezer for at least an hour.

Popsicles with almond milk and green tea

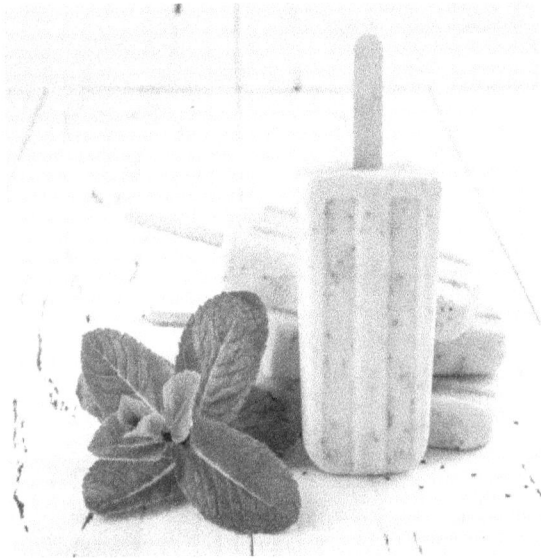

Pour the mixture into the appropriate containers or small paper coffee cups and place in the freezer for at least 2 hours.

At the time of serving, dip the containers in hot water for about 30 seconds, so you can easily remove the popsicles without tearing the stick.

Ingredients for 5 popsicles:

~ 300 ml almond (or rice) milk.
~ 3-4 tablespoons of rice malt
~ 1 teaspoon of green tea
~ 1 tablespoon of white almond cream
~ 1 pinch of whole sea salt

Instructions

Heat the milk and steep the tea for a few minutes.

Strain the milk and add the malt, pinch of salt and almond cream.

I suggest you give it a short whisk to mix well the almond cream that we need to add a fat component to the mixture and get a softer consistency. If instead you like more the typical texture of the popsicle, do not put the almond cream.

Crepes with pears and red fruits

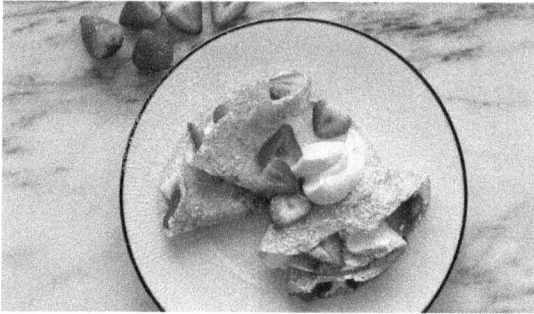

Ingredients for 4 crepes of 15 cm in diameter

- ~ 120 g of flour type 1 or 2 (semi wholemeal)
- ~ 150 ml of water
- ~ 1 pinch of turmeric (optional)
- ~ integral sea salt
- ~ 3 small pears
- ~ 200 g of red fruits (fresh or frozen)
- ~ 2 tablespoons of rice malt
- ~ extra virgin olive or sesame oil

Instructions

Peel the pears and cut them into cubes. Transfer them to a frying pan or saucepan with 2-3 tablespoons of water and a pinch of salt and cook for a few minutes until soft.

In another pan put the red berries with the malt. I used a mixture of raspberries and currants, but you can use just raspberries for example. If you use fresh fruit, add a little water as well. Let it cook for a few minutes while stirring.

Mix the flour with a pinch of salt and turmeric (it's for yellow colouring). Gradually add the water, stirring well with a whisk. You should get a fairly liquid batter.

Heat a non-stick pan greased with oil (I use a pan with a 15 cm diameter bottom).

When hot, pour in a ladleful of batter and move the pan to distribute the mixture well.

Cook a minute and turn the crepe with the help of a paddle. Cook the other side well and set aside. Prepare the others and when they are ready, stuff with the cooked pears. Close the crepes and pour the red fruits on top.

Crumbly cookies

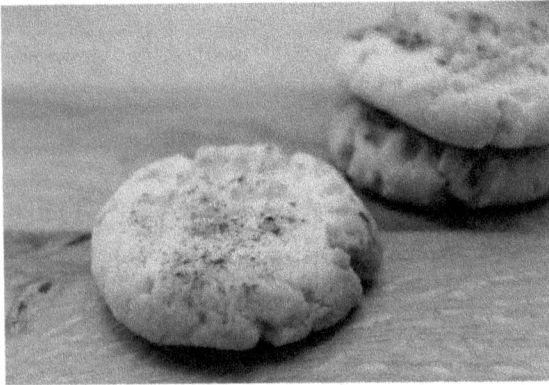

Ingredients for about 10 cookies

- ~ 1 tablespoon of chestnut flour
- ~ 1 tablespoon of rice flour
- ~ 2 tablespoons of cornstarch
- ~ 1 tablespoon of corn flour
- ~ 3 tablespoons flour type 1 or 2 or whole wheat flour
- ~ 3 tablespoons whole cane sugar (muscobado)
- ~ 1 tablespoon almond cream
- ~ 3-4 tablespoons of corn oil
- ~ 1 pinch of integral sea salt
- ~ vegetable milk

For the almond heart

- ~ 1 tablespoon almond cream (or hazelnut)
- ~ 2 tablespoons muscobado

For the accompanying milk:

- ~ 1 cup vegetable milk
- ~ 1 tablespoon malt
- ~ star anise
- ~ 1 pinch of turmeric

Instructions

Combine the flours, starch, salt and sugar and add the oil. Knead and form a ball. If needed, add a little vegetable milk or more oil. Wrap the ball in plastic wrap and let it rest in the refrigerator for half an hour.

Prepare the "heart" by combining the almond cream with the sugar.

Roll out the dough to a thickness of just under 1 cm and cut it as you prefer to make cookies.

Gently transfer them onto a baking sheet lined with parchment paper and with the tip of your finger make a small groove in the center of each cookie and deposit a small ball of almond cream.

Bake for 15 minutes at 170°.

Remove from the oven and leave to cool.

If you want to accompany them with aniseed and turmeric milk, transfer the milk to a small saucepan. Add the malt, turmeric and a star anise seed.

Bring to a boil while stirring and turn off.

Pumpkin and Raisin Biscuits

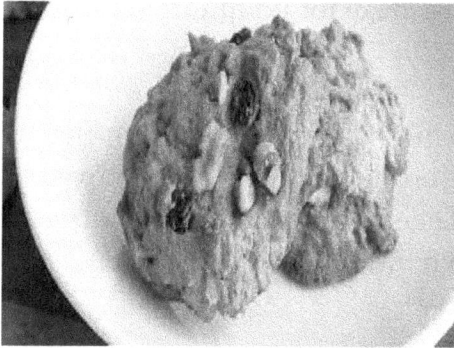

Ingredients

- ~ 150 g of wholemeal or semi-wholemeal spelt flour
- ~ 100 g of brown rice flour (if you do not have rice flour you can use another kind)
- ~ 300 g of cleaned pumpkin
- ~ 40 g of raisins
- ~ 60 g of evo oil
- ~ 1 heaped tablespoon of rice malt
- ~ 2 drops of verbena essential oil (just one may be enough)
- ~ 1 pinch of whole sea salt

Instructions

Slice or dice the pumpkin and bake it in the oven wrapped in aluminium foil for about 20 minutes at 180°. Take it out of the oven and let it cool a bit, then mash it with a fork until it becomes a puree.

Meanwhile, soak the raisins. In a bowl, combine the flours, salt and oil. Rub the flour between your hands so that it combines well with the oil.

Add the pumpkin puree, squeezed raisins, malt and verbena essential oil. I recommend no more than 2 drops! Knead quickly. If the dough is too hard add a little apple juice, if it is too soft add a little flour. Form a ball, wrap it in plastic wrap and refrigerate for an hour.

At this point roll out the dough and cut the cookies in the shapes you prefer.

Bake at 180 degrees for 15 minutes.

Soft cereal bars

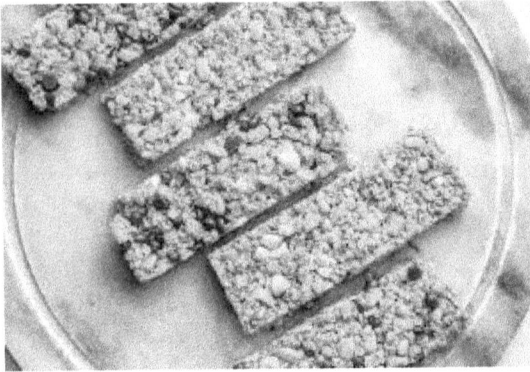

Ingredients

- ~ 4 tablespoons of cereal flakes (oats, barley, etc.)
- ~ 4 tablespoons of puffed cereals (rice, barley, spelt, quinoa, etc.)
- ~ 3 tablespoons of raisins
- ~ 3-4 dried apricots
- ~ 3-4 pieces of dried pears
- ~ 2 handfuls of hazelnuts
- ~ 2 tablespoons of sesame seeds
- ~ 3 tablespoons of rice malt
- ~ 50 of almonds reduced to flour
- ~ 150 g of dark chocolate (optional)

Instructions

Combine cereal flakes, raisins and dehydrated fruit in a bowl and cover with water to soften. In another bowl mix the puffed cereal with the sesame, chopped hazelnuts, almond flour and malt.

Squeeze out the ingredients that were soaking well and add them to the mixture. Mix well, mashing with a spoon.

Line a baking dish with baking paper and pour the mixture. Distribute it well, crushing and levelling. Bake for 30 minutes at 160°.

Meanwhile, melt the chocolate that you will pour over the mixture once removed from the oven. Let cool and place in the refrigerator for half an hour.

Remove the mixture with all the baking paper and turn it out onto a cutting board. Remove the paper and cut into bars.

This recipe lends itself to a thousand variations. I used apricots and pears, but you can also use other types of dehydrated fruit.

Castagnaccio

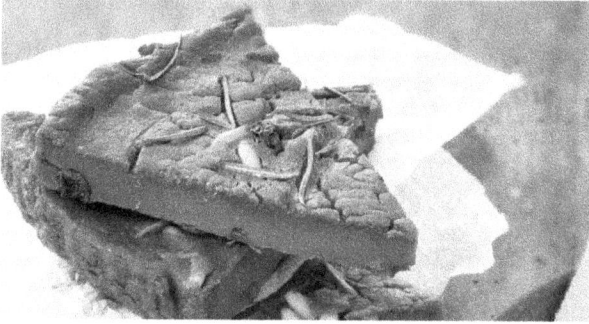

Add the pine nuts and rosemary leaves to the surface. Bake for about 40-45 minutes at 160°.

Ingredients

~ 300 g of chestnut flour
~ 300 ml of unsweetened vegetable milk
~ 200 ml of water
~ 2 tablespoons of extra virgin olive oil
~ 1 sprig of rosemary
~ 40 g of pine nuts
~ 50-60 g of raisins
~ 1-2 tablespoons of rice malt (optional)
~ 1 pinch of integral sea salt

Instructions

Chestnut flour tends to make lumps, so it's best to sift it.

Then add the salt, oil and a little at a time the milk and water, mixing well.

Add the raisins and, if you want to make a rather sweet chestnut cake, the malt.

Line a cake pan with baking paper, pour the mixture and arrange the raisins with a spoon so that they are evenly distributed.

Muffins with organic chocolate

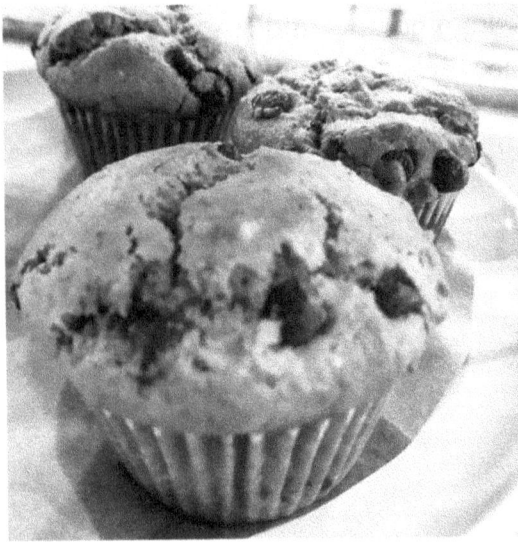

become liquid and mix well with the mixture. When melted, add it to the mixture.

Add the oil and a little at a time the milk to obtain a very soft consistency, almost liquid.

Using a spoon, transfer the mixture to the muffin cups, filling them about 3/4 full. I suggest you put the ramekins in a muffin mold right away to keep them in shape and then fill them. Bake at 160° for about 20 minutes.

Let cool well before serving.

Ingredients for 6 muffins:

~ 120 g semi whole wheat flour type 1 or type 2
~ 30 g of rice starch or arrowroot
~ 1 tablespoon of bitter cocoa
~ 50 g of dark chocolate (I used Quetzal with whole muscobado)
~ 60-70 g of Muscobado whole cane sugar (or 120 g of rice malt)
~ 1/2 sachet of cream of tartar natural yeast
~ 1/2 teaspoon of vanilla powder
~ 25 g of evo oil
~ 150 ml of unsweetened soy or oat milk
~ 1 pinch of whole sea salt

Instructions

Mix the flours, salt, cocoa, sugar, vanilla, baking powder and mix well.

Melt the chocolate in a bain-marie. The chocolate I used required a bit of soy milk to

Coconut rice cakes

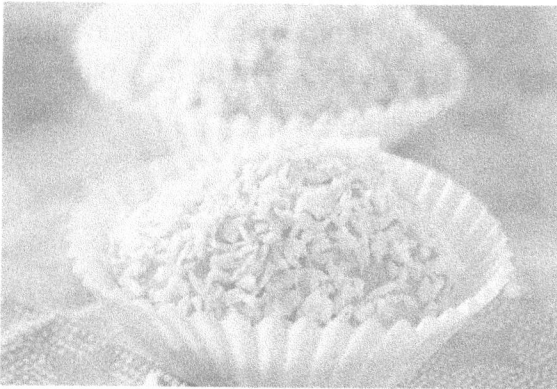

Cut dehydrated fruit into small pieces and add to rice. Add the malt and almond flour enough to make a moldable mixture (you may not need it, depending on how well the rice dries during cooking).

With wet hands shape into small balls and roll them in the coconut or in the almonds or hazelnuts or pistachios grains.

Refrigerate for half an hour before serving.

Ingredients for 15-20 treats:

~ 100 g brown rice
~ 300-350 ml almond milk (or water)
~ 1/2 vanilla stick
~ 1 pinch of whole sea salt
~ 3 tablespoons of rice malt (optional)
~ 100-150 g of dehydrated fruit to taste including raisins, apricots, pears, dates, figs, etc..
~ About 50-100 g of almonds reduced to flour
~ 100 g of coconut rapè

Instructions

Wash the rice and let it soak for 6-8 hours. Toss the water and cook it with the milk, vanilla bean stick and salt for about 30-35 minutes from boiling, partially covered.

By the end of cooking, the milk will be almost completely absorbed. Remove the vanilla stick and let cool covered. Incise the vanilla bean stick lengthwise and scoop out the seeds, which you can add to the cooked rice.

Strawberry Kanten

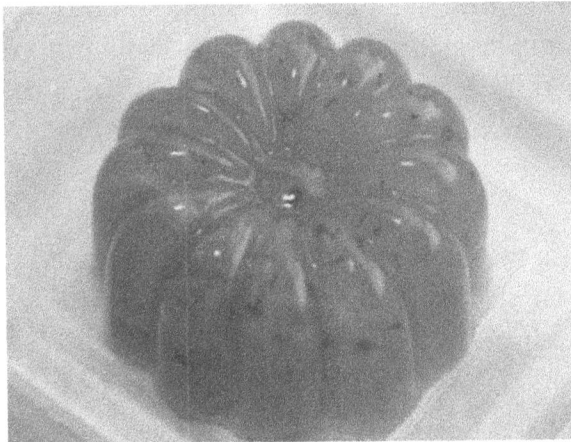

You can serve the kanten by themselves or you can accompany them with a few spoonfuls of chopped strawberries wilted in a pan with a little clear apple juice.

Ingredients for 4-6 small kanten:

- ~ 250 g ripe strawberries
- ~ 200 ml unsweetened soy or oat milk
- ~ 100 g of white soy yogurt
- ~ 2 level teaspoons of agar agar powder (about 4 g)
- ~ 4 tablespoons of rice malt
- ~ 1 pinch of whole sea salt

For the garnish:

- ~ 7-8 strawberries
- ~ 4-5 tablespoons of clear apple juice

Instructions

Clean the strawberries and cut them in half. Cook them in a small saucepan with the milk, malt, agar agar and salt for 5 minutes, stirring, until soft.

Whisk everything with the yogurt and transfer to molds.

Let cool and refrigerate for an hour or so.

Pear and almond cream

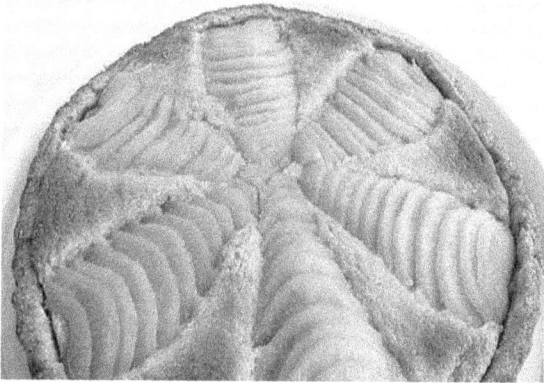

Ingredients

- ~ 500 ml of unsweetened oat or soy milk
- ~ 200 g of almonds
- ~ 200 g of rice malt
- ~ 2 ripe pears
- ~ 5 g of agar agar powder (about 2 heaped teaspoons)
- ~ 1 vanilla stick
- ~ 1 pinch of whole sea salt

Instructions

Reduce the almonds to flour, transfer to a blender and blend with the milk, agar agar, salt, pears and malt.

Transfer to a small saucepan, add the vanilla bean and bring to a boil, stirring constantly. Cook 1-2 minutes from a boil. Remove the vanilla bean, cut into it, scoop out the seeds and add to the mixture, stirring well. Let cool and transfer to the refrigerator until solidified.

Once the jelly has formed, whisk well to obtain a smooth cream and serve to taste accompanied by dark chocolate chips.

Rolling Coconut Truffles

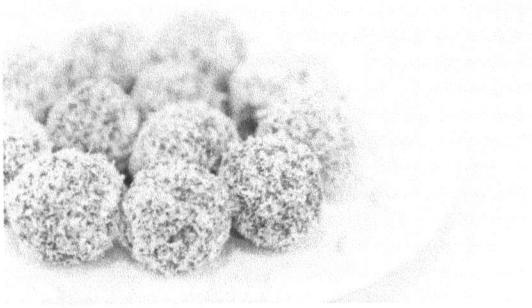

Ingredients

- ~ 140 g of fresh grated or blended coconut
- ~ 100 g of almonds
- ~ 2 tablespoons of rice malt
- ~ 2 teaspoons of mirin (optional)
- ~ bitter cocoa

Instructions

Add the pulverized almonds, malt and mirin to the blended or grated pulp. If you don't have mirin, you can use a little apple juice or a dessert liqueur.

Mix well and form small balls with your hands, then roll them in cocoa.

If the dough is too soft adding a little more ground almonds, if it is too hard adding a little apple juice or malt.

Tiramisù

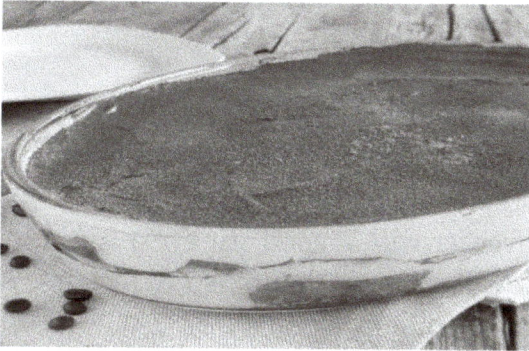

Ingredients for the sponge cake

- ~ 200 g semi-whole wheat flour type 2
- ~ 100 g of brown rice flour
- ~ 250 g of rice malt
- ~ 100 ml unsweetened soy or oat milk
- ~ 50 g of evo oil
- ~ 120 ml of apple juice
- ~ ½ sachet of cream of tartar natural yeast (about 9 g)
- ~ 1 teaspoon of vanilla powder
- ~ 1 pinch integral sea salt

For the pudding

- ~ 500 ml unsweetened almond milk (or other vegetable milk)
- ~ 20 g of bitter cocoa
- ~ 20 g brown rice flour
- ~ 4 g of agar-agar
- ~ 150 g of rice malt
- ~ 1 pinch of whole sea salt

For the accompanying cream

- ~ 200 ml unsweetened almond milk (or other vegetable milk)
- ~ 2 tablespoons of brown rice flour
- ~ 2 tablespoons of rice malt
- ~ 1 pinch of whole sea salt
- ~ Apple juice or mirin or cereal coffee (to soak the sponge cake once ready)

Prepare the sponge cake:

Mix the flours with the salt, vanilla and baking powder. Add the malt, oil and mix well. Slowly add the apple juice and soy milk. The dough should be quite liquid.

Pour the mixture into a baking pan lined with parchment paper and bake in a hot oven at 170 degrees for about 45 minutes. At the end of cooking let it cool well.

Prepare the cream:

Mix the flour with a little milk and add the cocoa, salt and agar-agar. Add the rest of the milk and bring to a boil while stirring. At the end of cooking add the rice malt and mix well until it is perfectly blended. Let cool and once cold whisk.

Prepare the cream:

Melt rice flour in a saucepan with a little almond milk, add the rest and salt and bring to a boil while stirring. Cook about 1 minute stirring. Transfer to a high bore container, add the malt and beat with an electric whisk for 1-2 minutes.

Compose the tiramisu:

Cut the sponge cake to your preferred thickness and size. Soak the sponge cake in the liquid of your choice and place it in the bottom of an oven dish or small cups. Add a layer of pudding and again the soaked sponge cake. The last layer will be pudding. Put in the refrigerator a couple of hours.

Chocolate and cinnamon ice cream

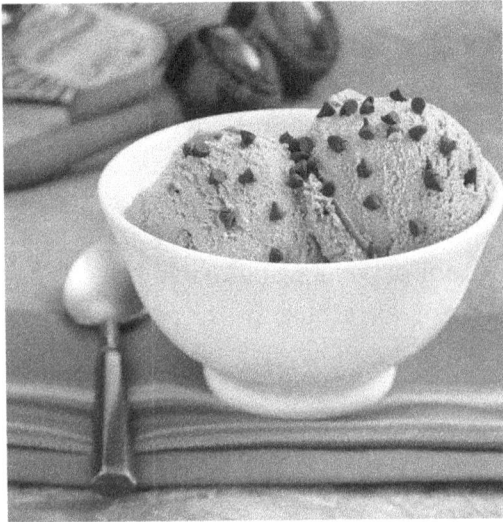

Ingredients

- ~ 300 g of unsweetened vegetable milk (rice, oats or almonds)
- ~ 3 tablespoons of almond or hazelnut cream
- ~ 150 g of dark chocolate
- ~ 1 cinnamon stick (or 1/2 teaspoon cinnamon powder)
- ~ 300 g of rice malt

Instructions

Bring the milk with the cinnamon stick to a boil and let it cool, then remove the cinnamon.

Break up the chocolate and melt it in a small saucepan with 2-3 tablespoons of milk. Add the rest of the milk a little at a time while stirring. Remove from heat and add the almond cream and malt. When cold pour into the ice cream maker and the vegan-macrobiotic ice cream is ready! If you wish you can decorate with chocolate chips or a sprinkling of cinnamon.

What if I don't have an ice cream maker?

No problem. The ice cream maker does nothing but cool and mix, continuously. We can replace it by simply alternating cooling in the freezer with a good stir every 30 minutes. This will take 4-5 hours, so 8-10 stirs. A bit tedious, but effective.

This operation is fundamental to chill the ice cream without the formation of ice crystals, so that it remains creamy. It is also convenient to pour the mixture into the already cold container.

Example Macrobiotic Diet

Secretary, does not play sports, and experiences continuous digestive system disturbances.

Sex
M

Age
44

Height cm
160

Wrist circumference cm
15,1

Constitution
Normal

Height/wrist
10,6

Morphological type
Normal

Weight kg
78

Body mass index
30,5

Desirable physiological body mass index
21,7

Desirable physiological weight kg
55,5

Basal Metabolism kcal
1312,3

Physical activity level coefficient
Light no aus, 1.42

Energy expenditure kcal
1863.5kcal

Hypochalor Diet - 30% 1304 Kcal
Breakfast 15% 196Kcal
Snack 5% 65Kcal
Lunch 40% 522Kcal
Snack 5% 65Kcal
Dinner 35% 456kcal

Day 1

Breakfast, about 15%kcal TOT

Boiled rice

Long grain brown rice, boiled   60g, 217,2kcal

Snack, about 5%kcal TOT

Dried walnuts   10g, 61,2kcal

Lunch, about 35%kcal TOT

Boiled Beans

Dried beans   100g, 311,0kcal

Wakame seaweed   200g, 90,0kcal

White bread   50g, 133,0kcal

Snack, about 5%kcal TOT

Almonds   10g, 57,5kcal

Dinner, about 35%kcal TOT

Boiled rice

Long grain brown rice, boiled   30g, 108,6kcal

Steamed chicken breast

Chicken breast, meat only	200g, 220,0kcal
Zucchinis, with skin	200g, 32,0kcal
White bread	25g, 66,5kcal

Day 2

Breakfast, about 15%kcal TOT

Boiled rice

Long grain brown rice, boiled	60g, 217,2kcal

Snack, about 5%kcal TOT

Pine nuts	10g, 62,9kcal

Lunch, about 35%kcal TOT

Boiled soybean

Dried soybeans	80g, 325,6kcal
Fennel, bulb	200g, 62,0kcal
White bread	50g, 133,0kcal

Snack, about 5%kcal TOT

Hazelnuts	10g, 62,8kcal

Dinner, about 35%kcal TOT

Boiled rice

Long grain brown rice, boiled	30g, 108,6kcal

Steamed Cod

Cod fillet	200g, 164,0kcal
Carrots	200g, 82,0kcal
White bread	25g, 66,5kcal

Day 3

Breakfast, about 15%kcal TOT

Boiled rice

Long grain brown rice, boiled	60g, 217,2kcal

Snack, about 5%kcal TOT

Pistachios	10g, 55,7kcal

Lunch, about 35%kcal TOT

Boiled chickpeas

Dried chickpeas	100g, 334,0kcal
Spinach	200g, 46,0kcal
White bread	50g, 133,0kcal

Snack, about 5%kcal TOT

Pecans	10g, 69,1kcal

Dinner, about 35%kcal TOT

Boiled rice

Long grain brown rice, boiled	30g, 108,6kcal

Tofu

Tofu	200g, 152,0kcal
Apple, with peel	200g, 104,0kcal
White bread	25g, 66,5kcal

Day 4

Breakfast, about 15%kcal TOT

Boiled rice

Long grain brown rice, boiled   60g, 217,2kcal

Snack, about 5%kcal TOT

Dried walnuts   10g, 61,2kcal

Lunch, about 35%kcal TOT

Boiled lentils

Dried lentils   100g, 325,0kcal

Wakame seaweed   200g, 90,0kcal

White bread   50g, 133,0kcal

Snack, about 5%kcal TOT

Almonds   10g, 57,5kcal

Dinner, about 35%kcal TOT

Boiled rice

Long grain brown rice, boiled   30g, 108,6kcal

Steamed sea bass

Sea bass fillet	250g, 205,0kcal
Mushrooms	200g, 40,0kcal
White bread	25g, 66,5kcal

Day 5

Breakfast, about 15%kcal TOT

    Boiled rice

    Long grain brown rice, boiled   60g, 217,2kcal

Snack, about 5%kcal TOT

    Pine nuts   10g, 62,9kcal

Lunch, about 35%kcal TOT

    Boiled soybean

        Dried soybeans   80g, 325,6kcal

    Fennel, bulb   200g, 62,0kcal

    White bread   50g, 133,0kcal

Snack, about 5%kcal TOT

    Hazelnuts   10g, 62,8kcal

Dinner, about 35%kcal TOT

    Boiled rice

        Long grain brown rice, boiled   30g, 108,6kcal

    Tempeh

Tempeh	100g, 193,0kcal
Carrots	200g, 82,0kcal
White bread	25g, 66,5kcal

Day 6

Breakfast, about 15%kcal TOT

Boiled rice

Long grain brown rice, boiled   60g, 217,2kcal

Snack, about 5%kcal TOT

Pistachios   10g, 55,7kcal

Lunch, about 35%kcal TOT

Boiled chickpeas

Dried chickpeas   100g, 334,0kcal

Spinach   200g, 46,0kcal

White bread   50g, 133,0kcal

Snack, about 5%kcal TOT

Pecans   10g, 69,1kcal

Dinner, about 35%kcal TOT

Boiled rice

Long grain brown rice, boiled   30g, 108,6kcal

Steamed fillet of sea bream

Sea bream	250g, 225,0kcal
Pear, peeled	200g, 116,0kcal
White bread	25g, 66,5kcal

Day 7

Breakfast, about 15%kcal TOT

Boiled rice

Long grain brown rice, boiled	60g, 217,2kcal

Snack, about 5%kcal TOT

Dried walnuts	10g, 61,2kcal

Lunch, about 35%kcal TOT

Boiled Beans

Dried beans	100g, 311,0kcal
Wakame seaweed	200g, 90,0kcal
White bread	50g, 133,0kcal

Snack, about 5%kcal TOT

Almonds	10g, 57,5kcal

Dinner, about 35%kcal TOT

Boiled rice

Long grain brown rice, boiled	30g, 108,6kcal

Tofu

Tofu	200g, 152,0kcal
Oranges	200g, 126,0kcal
White bread	25g, 66,5kcal

APPENDIX

Cooking Conversion Charts

INGREDIENTS	CONVERSION US	CONVERSION EU
cup	16 tablespoons	236 ml
fluid ounce – fl.oz.	–	30 ml
pinch / dash	1/16 teaspoon	–
pint	2 cups	0,47 l
pound	16 ounces	454 g
quart	4 cups	0,95 l
teaspoon – tsp	1/3 tablespoon	5 ml
tablespoon – tbsp	3 teaspoons	15 ml
ounce – oz	–	28 g

Dry Ingredients

INGREDIENTS	CONVERSION
Cake/Pastry Flour	1 cup : 115 g
All-purpose	1 cup : 125 g
High gluten	1 cup : 140 g
Whole wheat	1 cup : 120 g
Bread flour	1 cup : 130 g
Spelt	1 cup : 100 g
Light Rye	1 cup : 100 g
Dark Rye	1 cup : 125 g
Buckweat	1 cup : 120 g
Rice	1 cup : 185 g
Sugar	1 cup : 200 g
Brown Sugar	1 cup : 220 g
Powdered Sugar	1 cup : 120 g
Baking Soda	1 tsp : 5 g
Baking Powder	1 tsp : 5 g
Fresh yeast	1 tsp : 3 g
Active dry yeast	1 tsp : 3 g
Salt	1 tbsp : 18 g
Chocolate chips	1 cup : 160 g
Cocoa	1 cup : 120 g

Fresh ingredients

INGREDIENTS	CONVERSIONS
Water	1 cup : 236 ml
Milk	1 cup : 245 ml
Yogurt	1 cup : 245 ml
Cream	1 cup : 245 ml
Buttermilk	1 cup : 245 ml
Olive Oil	• 1 cup : 222 ml • 1 tbsp : 13 g
Butter	• 1 cup : 230 g • 1 tbsp : 14.5 g • 1 stick : 1/2 cup : 8 tbsp : 115 g
Eggs	1 cup : 275 g
(Egg) Whites	1 cup : 240 g
(Egg) Yolks	1 cup : 300 g
Honey	• 1 cup : 340 g • 1 tbsp : 20 g
Grated cheese	1 cup : 110 g
Vanilla extract	1 tsp : 4 g
Peanut Butter	1 cup : 258 g

Oven Temperatures

250 °F	120 °C
275 °F	140 °C
300 °F	150 °C
325 °F	160 °C
350 °F	180 °C
375 °F	190 °C
400 °F	200 °C
425 °F	220 °C
450 °F	230 °C
475 °F	240 °C
500 °F	260 °C